More
Than
a Scar

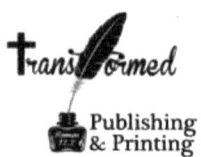

Mission: To Proclaim Transformation and Truth
Publisher: Transformed Publishing, Cocoa, FL
Website: www.transformedpublishing.com
Email: transformedpublishing@gmail.com

ISBN: 978-1-953241-76-4 (paperback)
ISBN: 978-1-953241-78-8 (hardcover)

Bonita Anderson

More Than a Scar

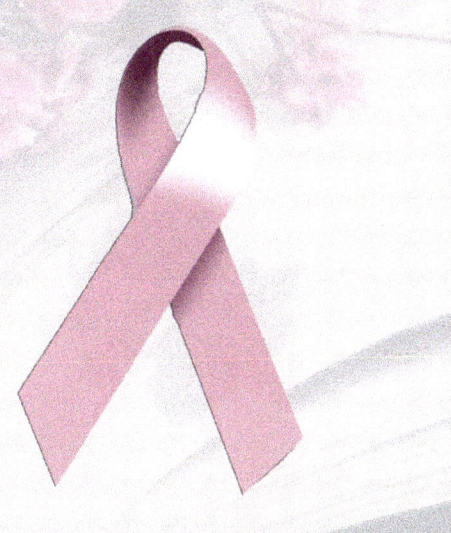

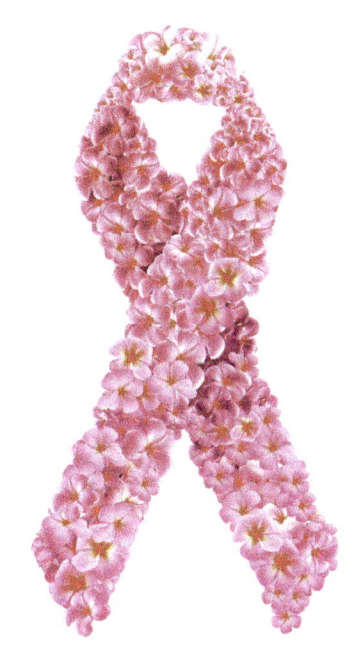

Yea, though I walk through the
valley of the shadow of death,
I will fear no evil;
For You *are* with me;
Your rod and Your staff,
they comfort me.
-Psalm 23:4

The purpose of this book is for you to JOURNAL YOUR JOURNEY OF EXPERIENCES

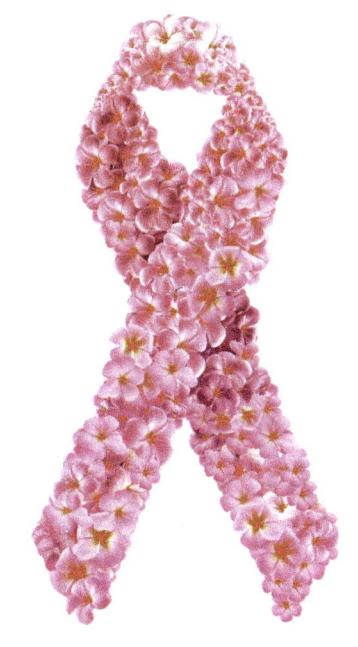

Foreword:

Written by Bonita's husband, Lester Anderson

Bonita Wright-Anderson is a Breast Cancer Survivor, devoted Christian, wife to Lester Anderson, and mother of four. She comes from a large family consisting of four brothers and many extended relatives. She was raised by a strong single mother in the western community of Pahokee, Florida out in the Glades. Her humble beginnings and deep devotion to her Christian faith helped to shape the woman she is today.

Bonita survived breast cancer in 2016 and has since dedicated her life to encouraging and guiding others through their own cancer journey, so they never have to face it alone. With over twenty years of experience as a registered nurse and nurse educator, she brings both professional, expertise, and personal insights to every page of her writing.

Bonita was honored in Palm Beach County as Lakeside Medical Center Nurse of the Year in 2017. Bonita served her community with distinction through her involvement in Delta Sigma Theta Sorority, Incorporated as chair of the Physical and Mental Health Committee from 2021 to 2023. With the help of Promise Fund of Florida, she successfully secured a $10,000 grant to provide free mammograms to residents of the Glades community reflecting her deep commitment to health equity and access.

This is her first published journal: a spirit-filled, encouraging resource inspired by her faith, her journey and her passion for supporting others. Bonita is known for her compassion, her unwavering love for Christ, and her dedication as a friend. I am sure this journal will allow you to in script your experiences and remember your why.

Table of Contents

Personal Story:
A Journey of Faith   1
Through Breast Cancer

Plan of Care
List of Your Doctors   5
& Important Dates

Summary of Diagnosis   6
& Pathology

Calendar of Care   8

Journey of Care   20

40 Day Journal of Care   23

Testimonies of Others   105

Your Personal Testimony   111

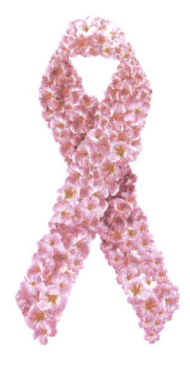

Personal Story:
A Journey of Faith Through Breast Cancer

On a late Thursday afternoon, after all the Operating Room (OR) cases were completed, I was called to an exam room by a coworker. There, the surgeon I work with every day gave me the news no one ever wants to hear:

"You have breast cancer."

I drove home in utter disbelief and shock. The car ride was quiet, my mind clouded with worry and fear. Thoughts raced: *Would I survive? Who would raise my children if I didn't make it?* In that moment, cancer felt like a death sentence.

It wasn't until I arrived home that I felt the Spirit whisper:

"Go into your prayer closet."

While there, I heard clearly:

**"You shall not die,
but live, and declare the works of the Lord."**
(*see* Psalm 118:17)

At that moment, every burden, every doubt, and every fear lifted. I felt a strength rise in me—a readiness to do whatever I needed to do to live.

At first, I didn't tell my family. I needed a plan before I shared the news with those I loved. However, I did tell my coworkers, knowing that my absence would affect them. We gathered in the nursing lounge, where emotions ran high as I shared the diagnosis. To lighten the mood, I joked with the housekeeper that I was secretly pregnant by the anesthesiologist! (A much-needed laugh in a heavy moment.)

That Monday, my manager had already taken initiative. She'd spoken to the Palm Beach Nurse Navigator for Breast Cancer and gathered all the information I would need. That preparation made the next steps much easier.

Once I had a clear plan, I informed my family. We created a support group to help me through appointments, treatments, and surgery.

God's Hand in Every Detail

God knows everything concerning us. Jeremiah 29:11 confirms that:

> **For I know the thoughts that I think toward you, says the Lord, thoughts of peace and not of evil, to give you a future and a hope.**

It was no coincidence that the very person who taught me to insert a PICC line (peripherally inserted central catheter) also survived breast cancer. My manager remembered her and reached out on my behalf. That divine connection guided me through the next steps of treatment.

After many appointments and tests, it was determined that I did *not* need chemotherapy—only radiation. Praise God!

My surgery was performed at Good Samaritan Hospital, and on the day of surgery, God placed someone at every encounter to remind me I was not alone:

- The transporter introduced himself as my "spiritual brother."
- Someone prayed for me just before surgery.

A coworker from Lakeside Medical Center who works at Good Samaritan met me at the MRI room, moments after a prayer call ended—another familiar face with a praying heart.

Even during the intense and uncomfortable MRI, God's presence was a calming balm. As an OR nurse myself, I felt comforted talking with the anesthesiologist just before surgery—a soothing way to fall asleep.

Recovery and Radiation

Eight weeks of recovery gave me time to rest, reconnect with family, and deepen my walk with God. The love I received during that time from my family, friends, coworkers, and church was overwhelming—a true reminder of how deeply I am loved.

Radiation began at SFRO (South Florida Radiation Oncology Center), where I underwent 32 rounds.

The staff was nothing short of amazing. I worked every day during treatment, scheduling sessions in the afternoon. And I never went alone—my mom, son, and daughter took turns driving me.

The first session was frightening—I had a panic attack. But then I remembered what a sister from church told me:

"Recite Psalm 23 every time you go for treatment."

And so I did. Each time, I would recite:

"The Lord is my shepherd…"

And I would fall asleep in peace. The technician even asked,

"What do you say before you fall asleep during treatment?"

Even during radiation, God gave me opportunities to witness and encourage other patients. He truly placed a support system around me every step of the way.

Today, I Am a Living Testimony

Hearing "you have breast cancer" felt like a death sentence—but I stand here today, a survivor and a witness to **God's goodness**.

Email: Bonita Anderson
morethanascar2016@gmail.com

Plan of Care
List of Your Doctors & Important Dates

Diagnosis:	
Pathology:	
Primary Diagnosis:	
Mammogram Facility / Date:	
Radiologist:	
Primary Doctor:	
Surgery Date:	
Surgeon:	
Radiation Oncologist:	
Chemo Diagnosis:	
Chemo Drug:	
Plastic Surgeon:	
Gynecologist:	

Summary
of Diagnosis & Pathology Reports

What have you been diagnosed with by the physician? What does the pathology report say?

Month / Year:

SUNDAY	MONDAY	TUESDAY	WEDNESDAY
___	___	___	___
___	___	___	___
___	___	___	___
___	___	___	___
___	___	___	___

Goal:

THURSDAY	FRIDAY	SATURDAY	NOTES:
___	___	___	
___	___	___	
___	___	___	
___	___	___	
___	___	___	

Month / Year:

SUNDAY	MONDAY	TUESDAY	WEDNESDAY
——	——	——	——
——	——	——	——
——	——	——	——
——	——	——	——
——	——	——	——

Goal:

THURSDAY	FRIDAY	SATURDAY	NOTES:
___	___	___	
___	___	___	
___	___	___	
___	___	___	
___	___	___	

Month / Year:

SUNDAY	MONDAY	TUESDAY	WEDNESDAY
——	——	——	——
——	——	——	——
——	——	——	——
——	——	——	——
——	——	——	——

Goal:

THURSDAY	FRIDAY	SATURDAY	NOTES:
___	___	___	
___	___	___	
___	___	___	
___	___	___	
___	___	___	

Month / Year:

SUNDAY	MONDAY	TUESDAY	WEDNESDAY
___	___	___	___
___	___	___	___
___	___	___	___
___	___	___	___
___	___	___	___

Goal:

THURSDAY	FRIDAY	SATURDAY	NOTES:
____	____	____	
____	____	____	
____	____	____	
____	____	____	
____	____	____	

Month / Year:

SUNDAY	MONDAY	TUESDAY	WEDNESDAY
___	___	___	___
___	___	___	___
___	___	___	___
___	___	___	___
___	___	___	___

Goal:

THURSDAY	FRIDAY	SATURDAY	NOTES:
_____	_____	_____	
_____	_____	_____	
_____	_____	_____	
_____	_____	_____	
_____	_____	_____	

Month / Year:

SUNDAY	MONDAY	TUESDAY	WEDNESDAY
___	___	___	___
___	___	___	___
___	___	___	___
___	___	___	___
___	___	___	___

Goal:

THURSDAY	FRIDAY	SATURDAY	NOTES:
___	___	___	
___	___	___	
___	___	___	
___	___	___	
___	___	___	

Journey of Care

A Place to Write About Your Care . . .

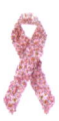

More Than a Scar

40 Day Journal of Care

Date: _____ # Day 1

Yea, though I walk through the valley
of the shadow of death, I will fear no evil:
for thou art with me; thy rod and
thy staff they comfort me.
-Psalm 23:4 KJV

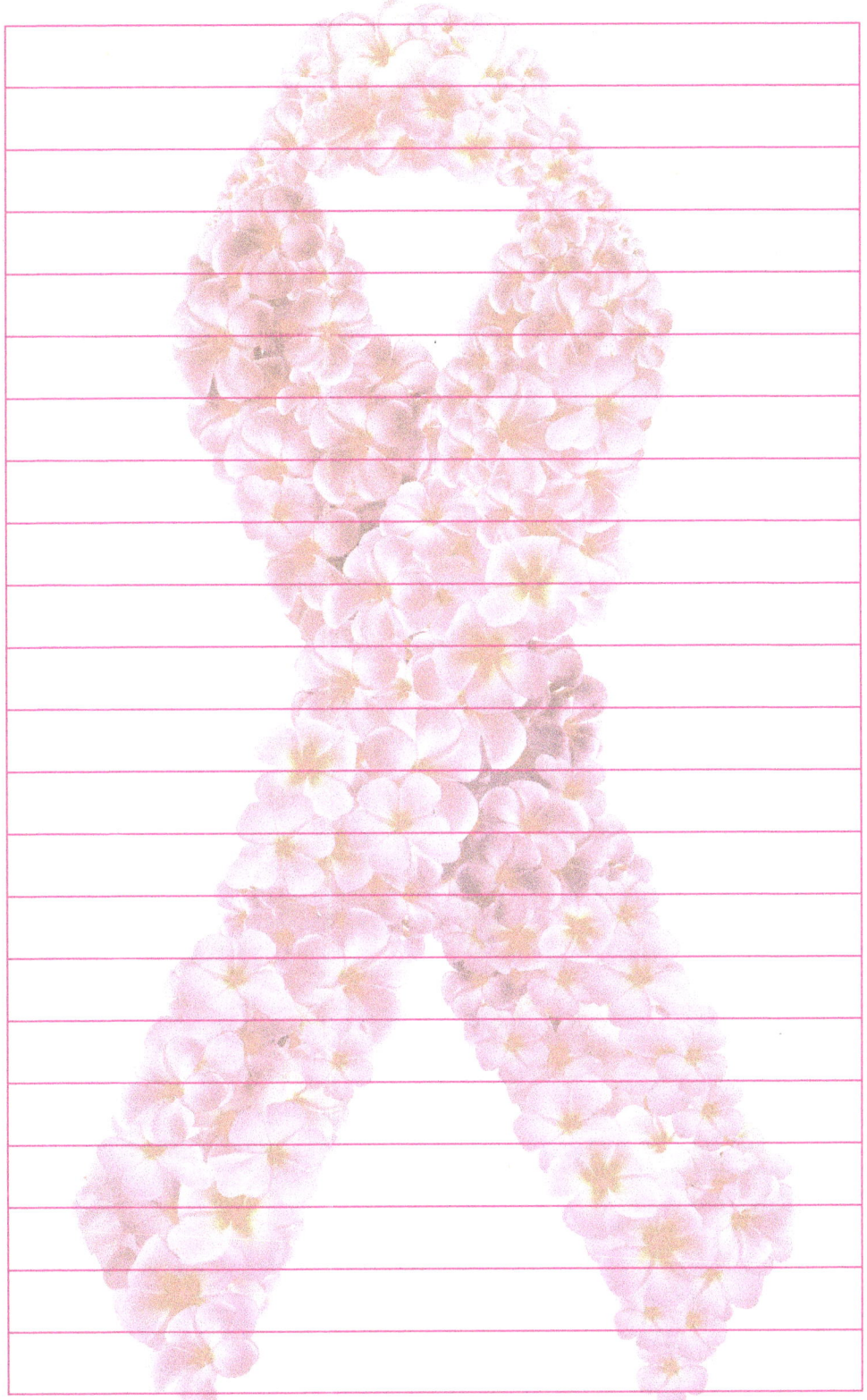

Date: _____ **Day 2**

Whoever dwells in the shelter
of the Most High will rest in the
shadow of the Almighty
-Psalm 91:1 NIV

Date: _____  **Day 3**

["]For I know the plans I have for you,"
declares the Lord, "plans to prosper
you and not to harm you, plans to
give you hope and a future.["]
-Jeremiah 29:11 NIV

Date: _____ 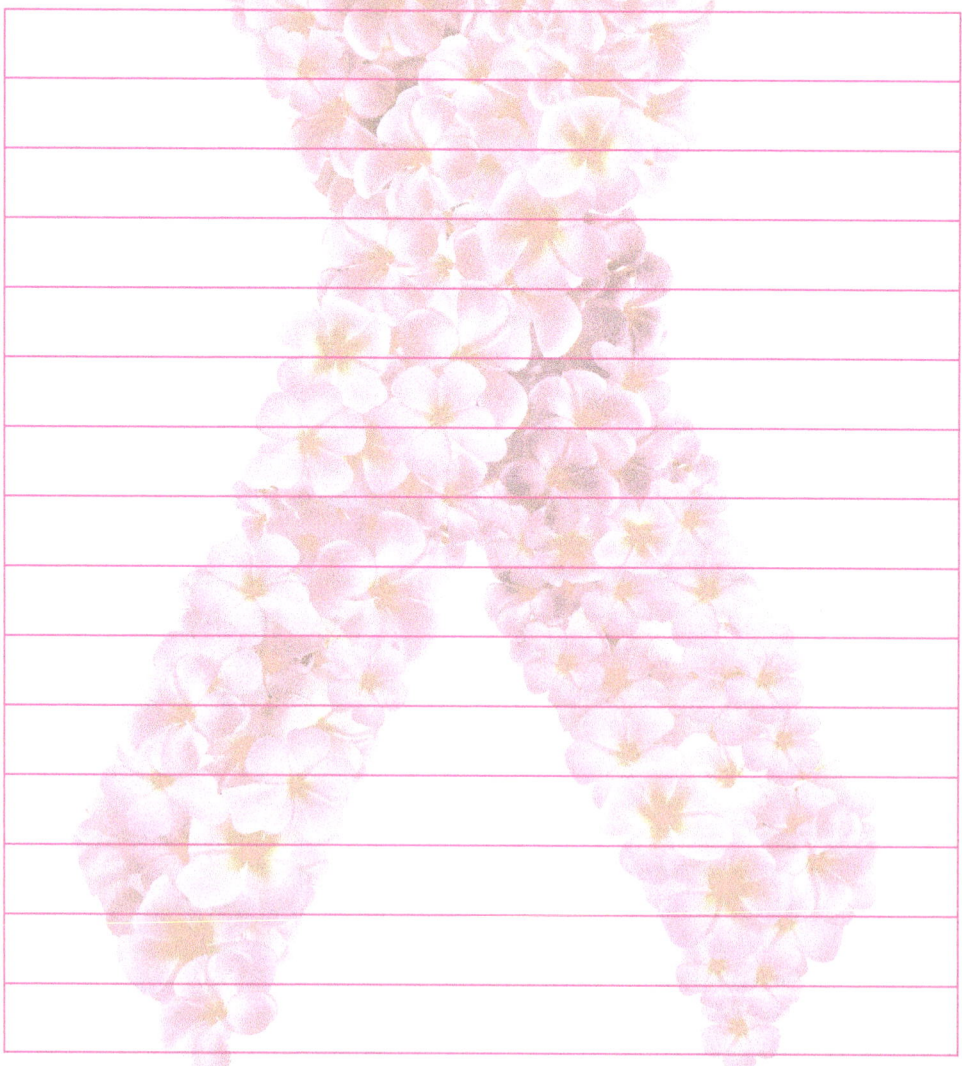 # Day 4

I shall not die, but live,
and declare the works of the Lord.
-Psalm 118:17 KJV

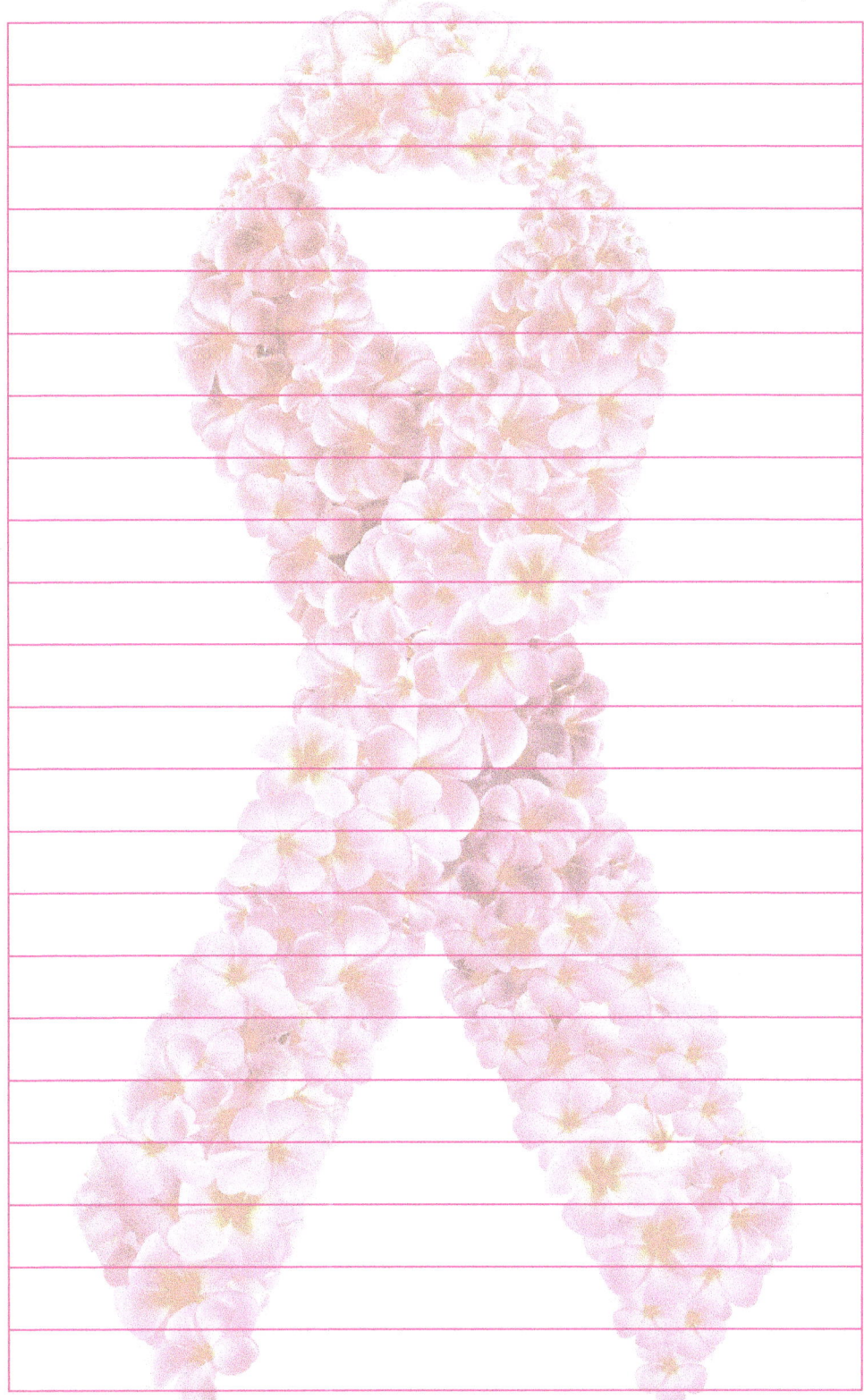

Date: _____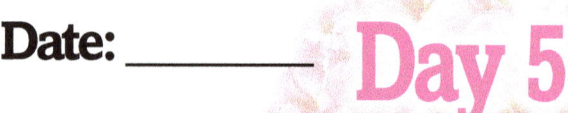

Fear not, O land; be glad and rejoice:
for the Lord will do great things.
-Joel 2:21 KJV

Date: _____ # Day 6

[B]eing confident of this, that he who began a good work in you will carry it on to completion until the day of Christ Jesus.
-Philippians 1:6 NIV

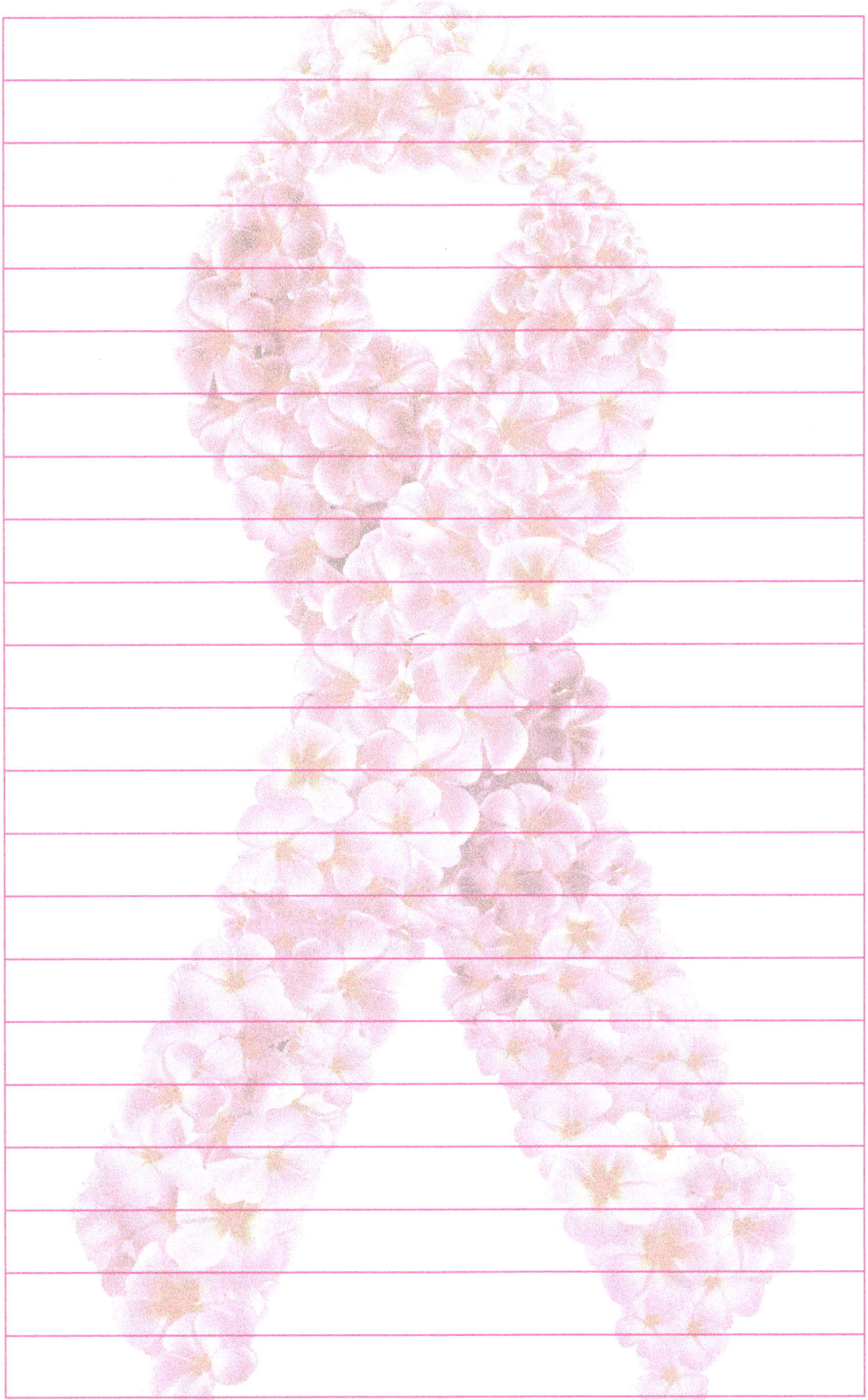

Date: _____ **Day 7**

"Do not be afraid, little flock,
for your Father has been pleased
to give you the kingdom.["]
-Luke 12:32 NIV

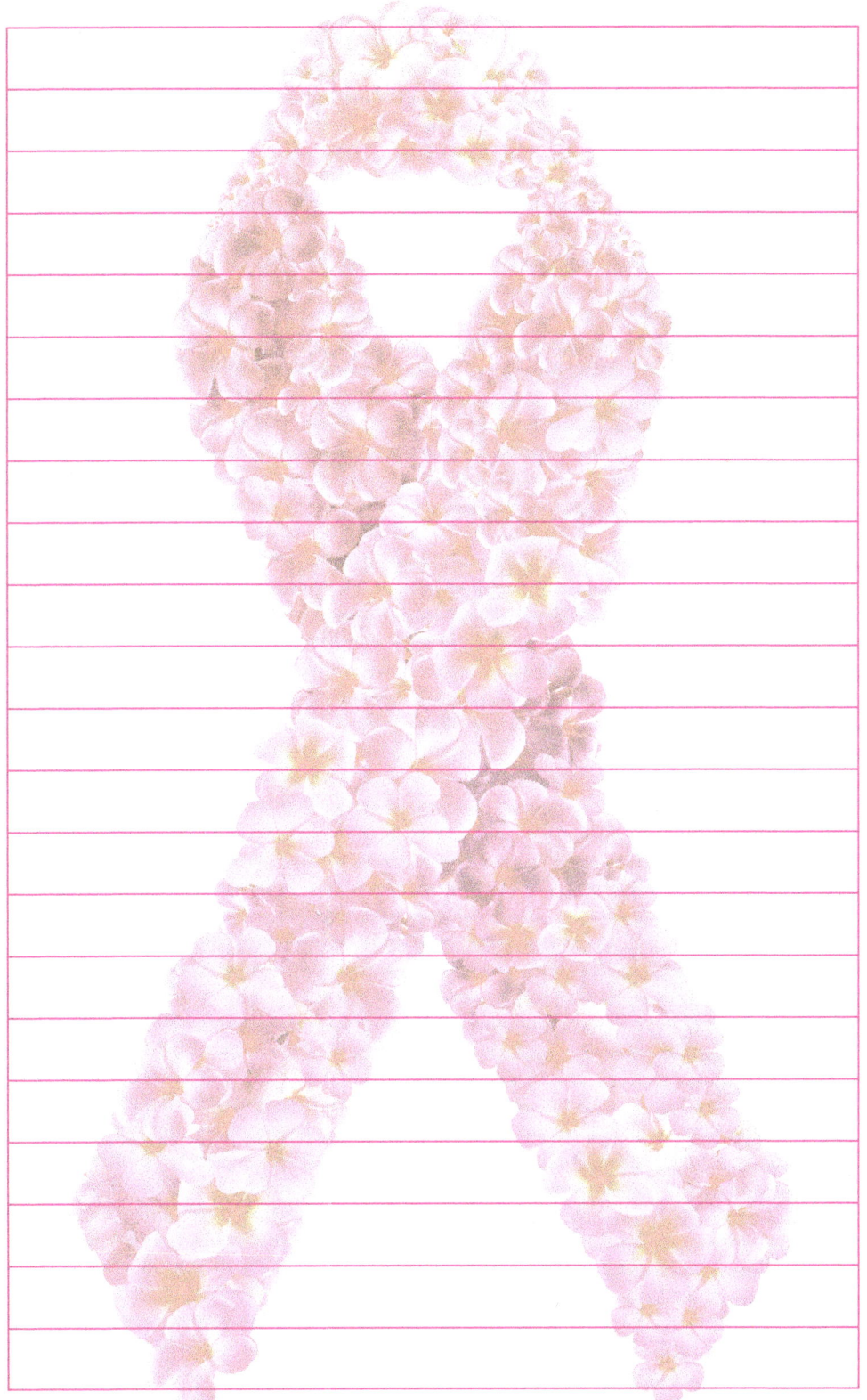

Date: _____ # Day 8

Do not be anxious about anything,
but in every situation, by prayer
and petition, with thanksgiving,
present your requests to God.
And the peace of God, which transcends
all understanding, will guard your hearts
and your minds in Christ Jesus.
-Philippians 4:6-7 NIV

Date: _____   **Day 9**

He says, "Be still, and know that I am God;
I will be exalted among the nations,
I will be exalted in the earth."
-Psalm 46:10 NIV

Date: _____ **Day 10**

["]Be strong and courageous.
Do not be afraid or terrified because
of them, for the Lord your God goes
with you; he will never leave
you nor forsake you."
-Deuteronomy 31:6 NIV

Date: _____ **Day 11**

Finally, my brethren, be strong in the Lord,
and in the power of his might.
-Ephesians 6:10 KJV

Date: _____ 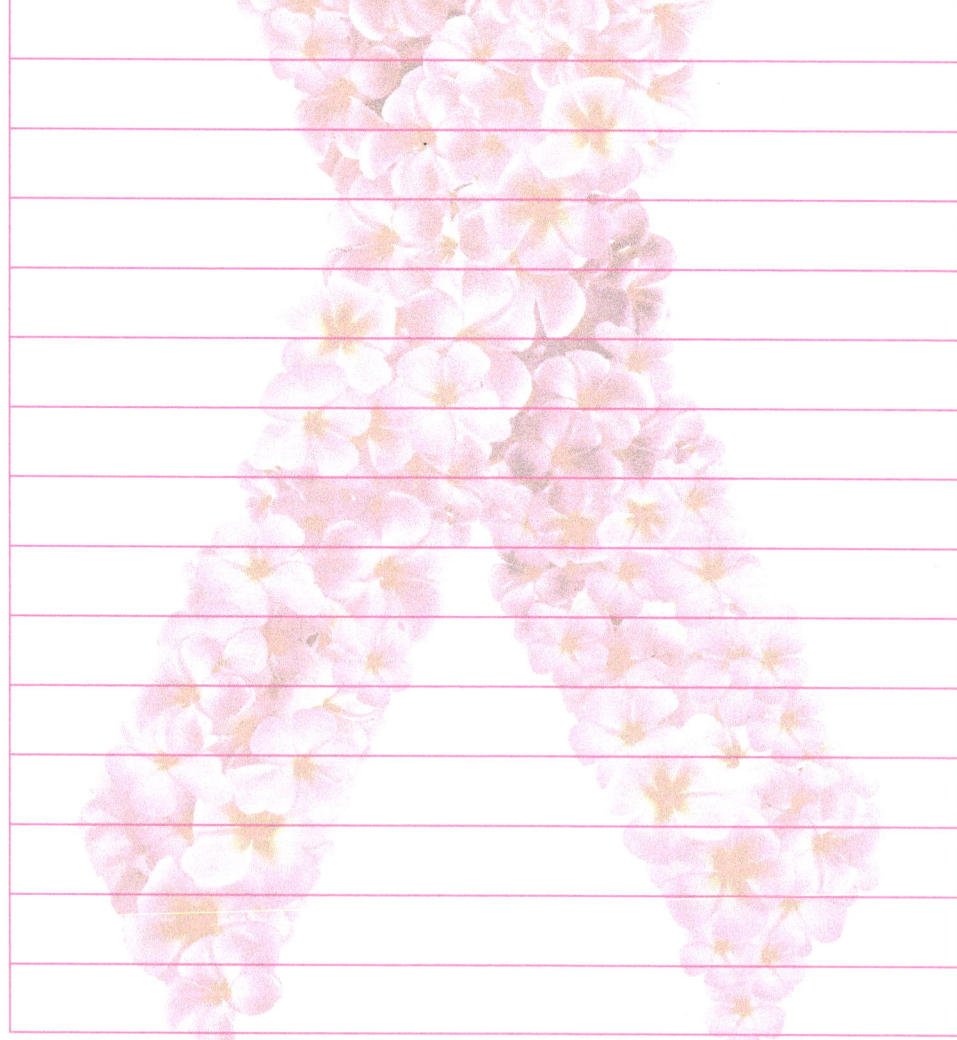 ## Day 12

God is our refuge and strength,
an ever-present help in trouble.
-Psalm 46:1 NIV

Date: _____ 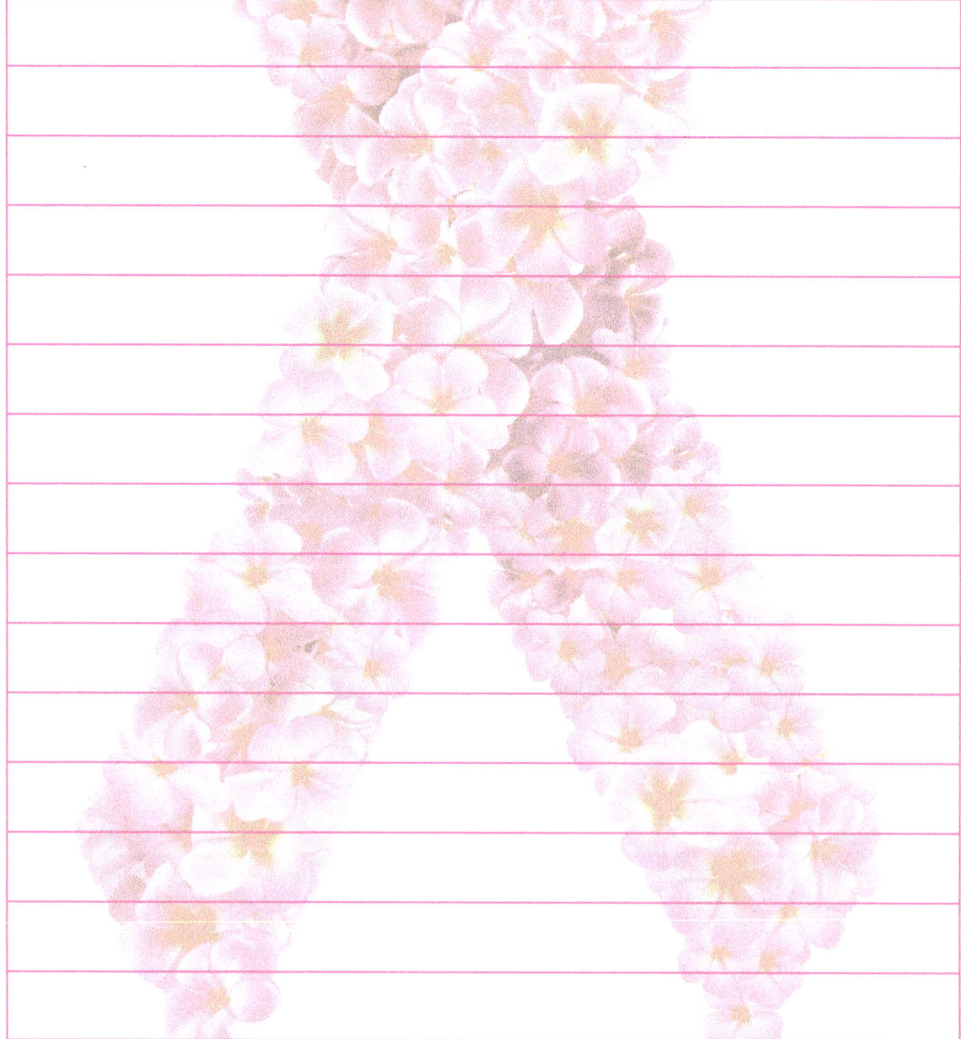 Day 13

A cheerful heart is good medicine,
but a crushed spirit dries up the bones.
-Proverbs 17:22 NIV

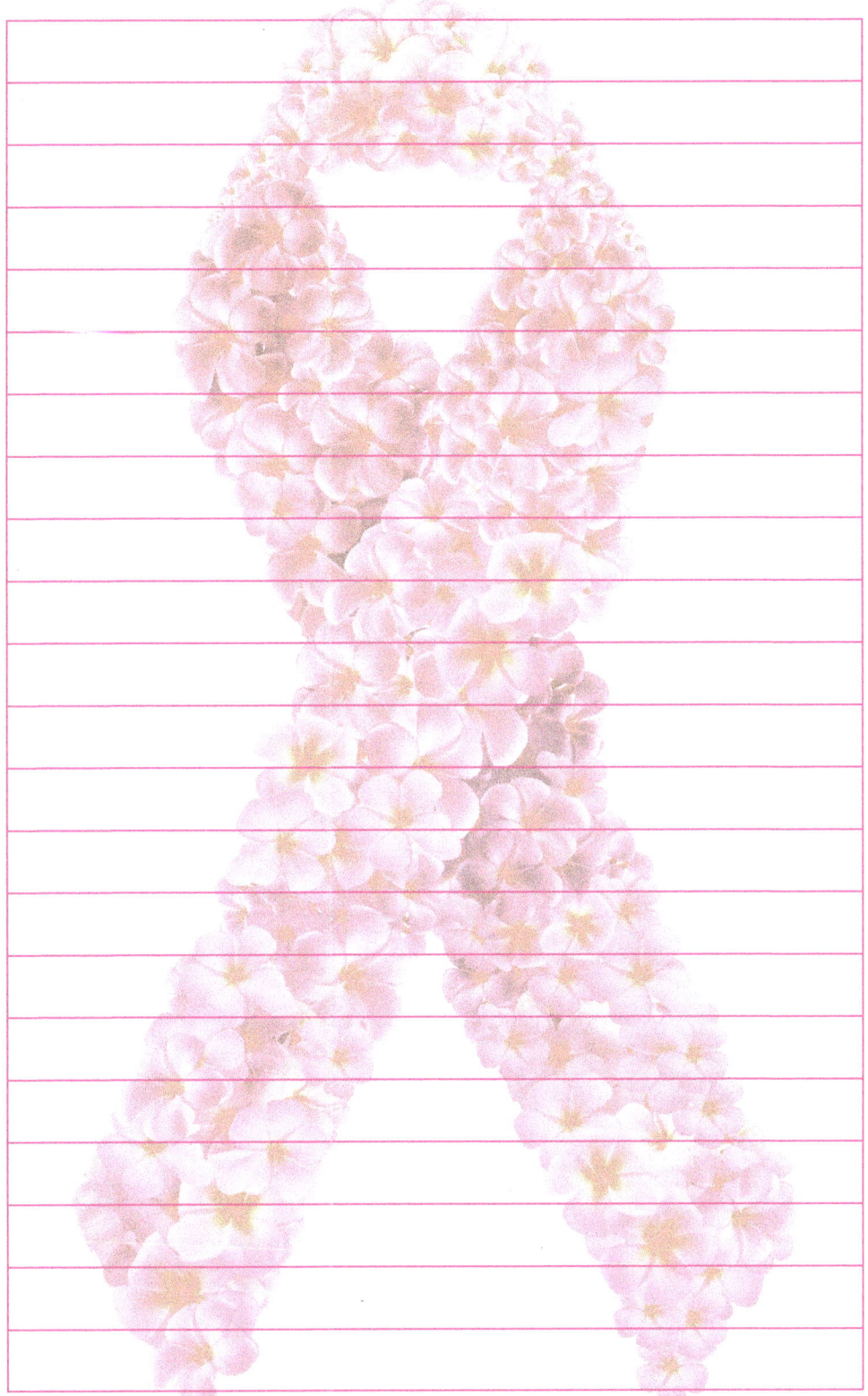

Date: _____ **Day 14**

I can do all this through him
who gives me strength.
-Philippians 4:13 NIV

Date: _____ **Day 15**

Beloved, I wish above all things that
thou mayest prosper and be in health,
even as thy soul prospereth.
-3 John 1:2 KJV

Date: _____ **Day 16**

So do not fear, for I am with you;
do not be dismayed, for I am your God.
I will strengthen you and help you;
I will uphold you with my
righteous right hand.
-Isaiah 41:10 NIV

Date: _____ **Day 17**

Now faith is confidence in what
we hope for and assurance
about what we do not see.
-Hebrews 11:1 NIV

Date: _____ **Day 18**

I keep my eyes always on the Lord.
With him at my right hand,
I will not be shaken.
-Psalm 16:8 NIV

Date: _____

Day 19

"I have told you these things,
so that in me you may have peace.
In this world you will have trouble.
But take heart! I have overcome the world."
-John 16:33 NIV

Date: _____ **Day 20**

For God hath not given us the spirit of fear,
but of power, and of love,
and of a sound mind.
-2 Timothy 1:7 KJV

Date: _____ 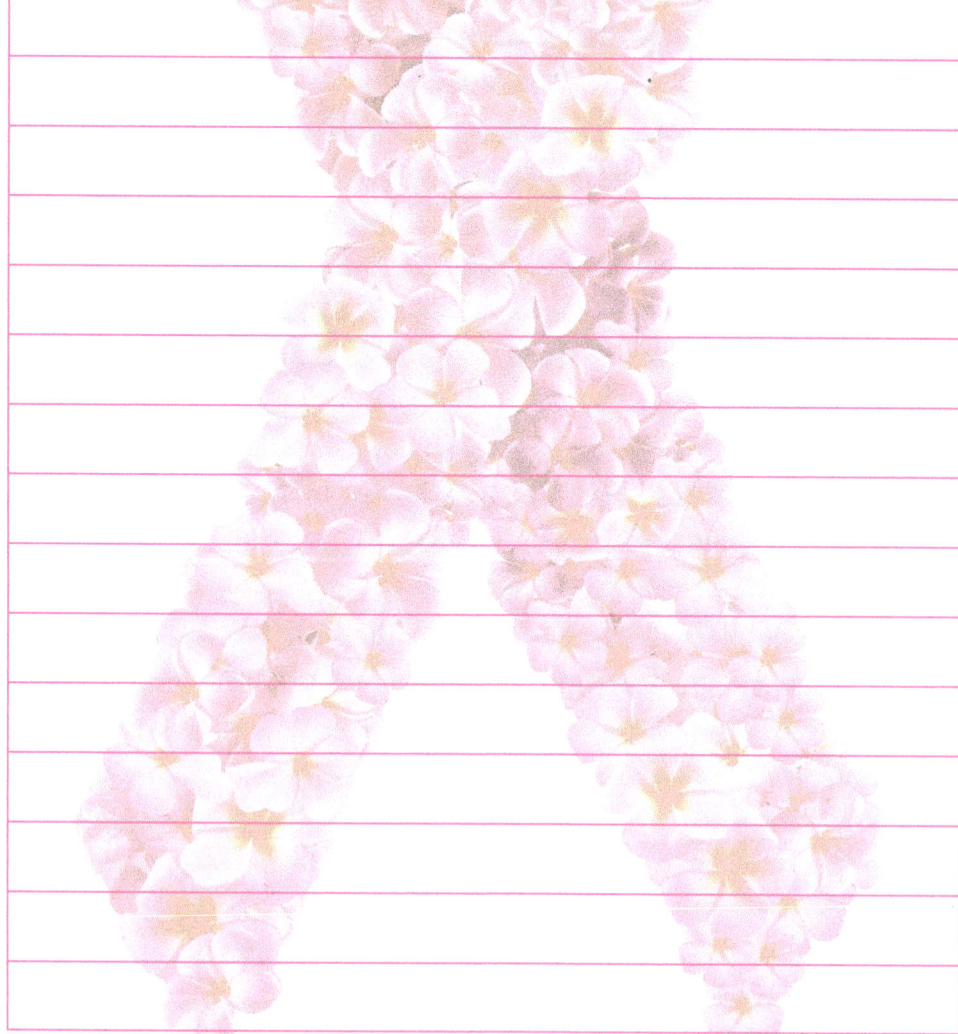 # Day 21

Let us not become weary in doing good,
for at the proper time we will reap
a harvest if we do not give up.
-Galatians 6:9 NIV

Date: _____ **Day 22**

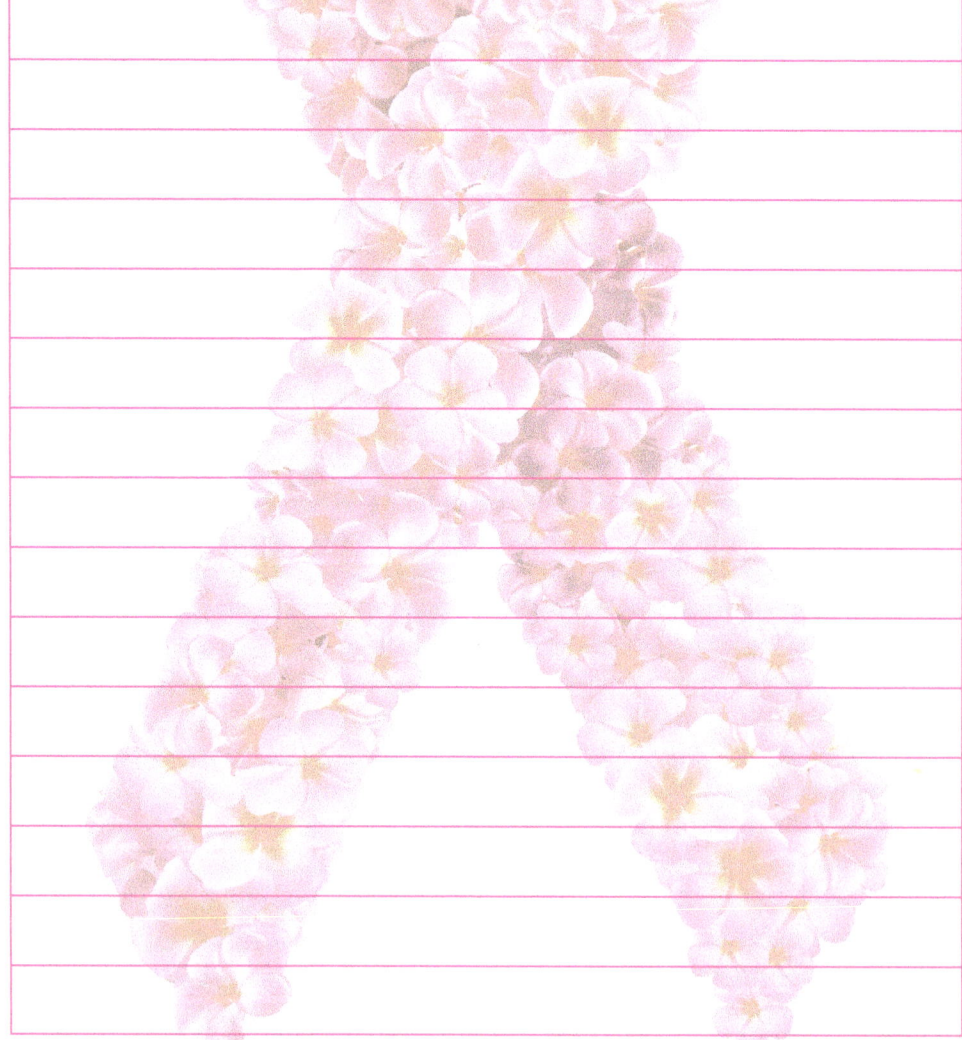

"Come to me, all you who are weary
and burdened, and I will give you rest."
-Matthew 11:28 NIV

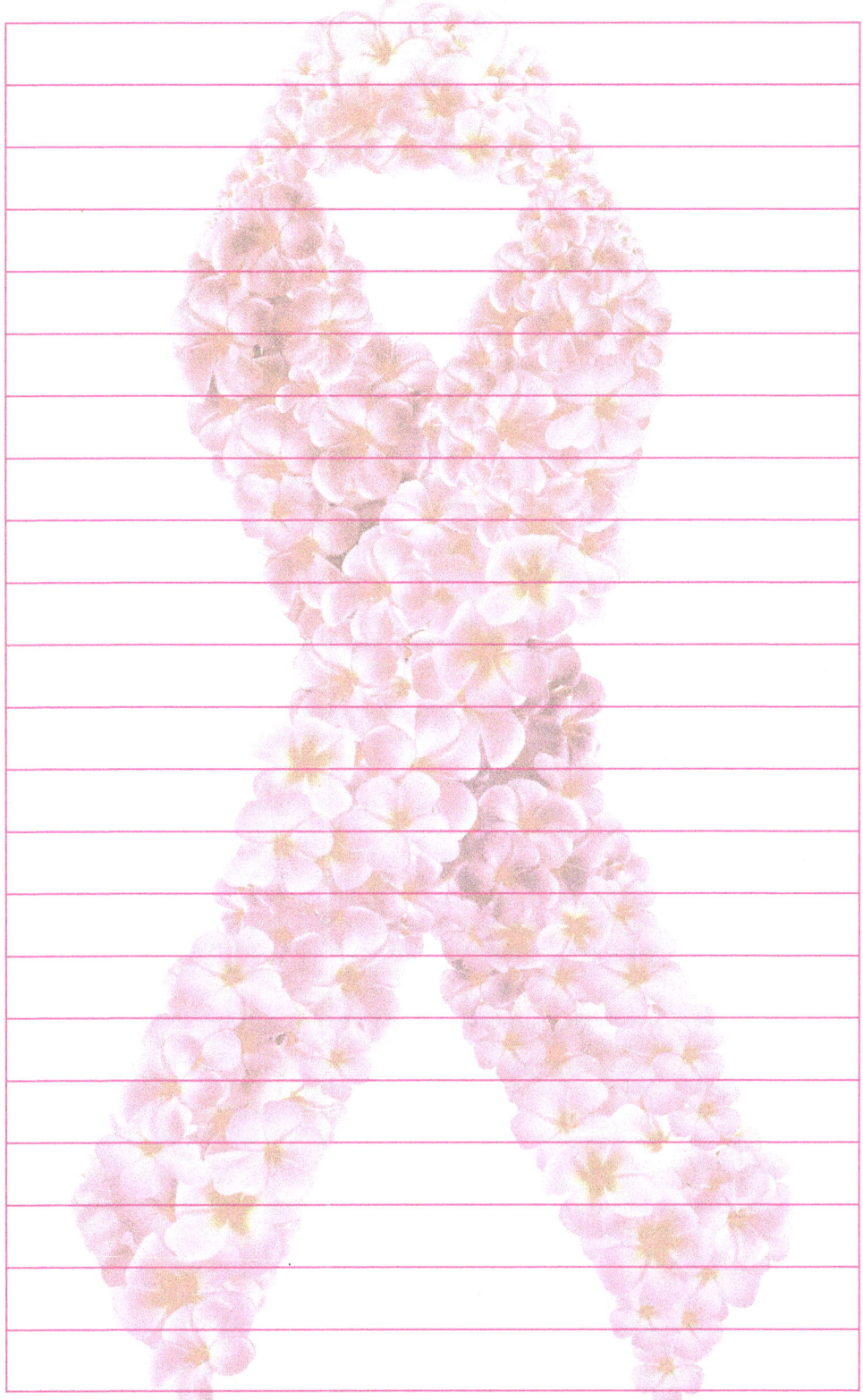

Date: _____ **Day 23**

My help comes from the Lord,
the Maker of heaven and earth.
-Psalm 121:2 NIV

Date: _____ **Day 24**

Heal me, Lord, and I will be healed;
save me and I will be saved,
for you are the one I praise.
-Jeremiah 17:14 NIV

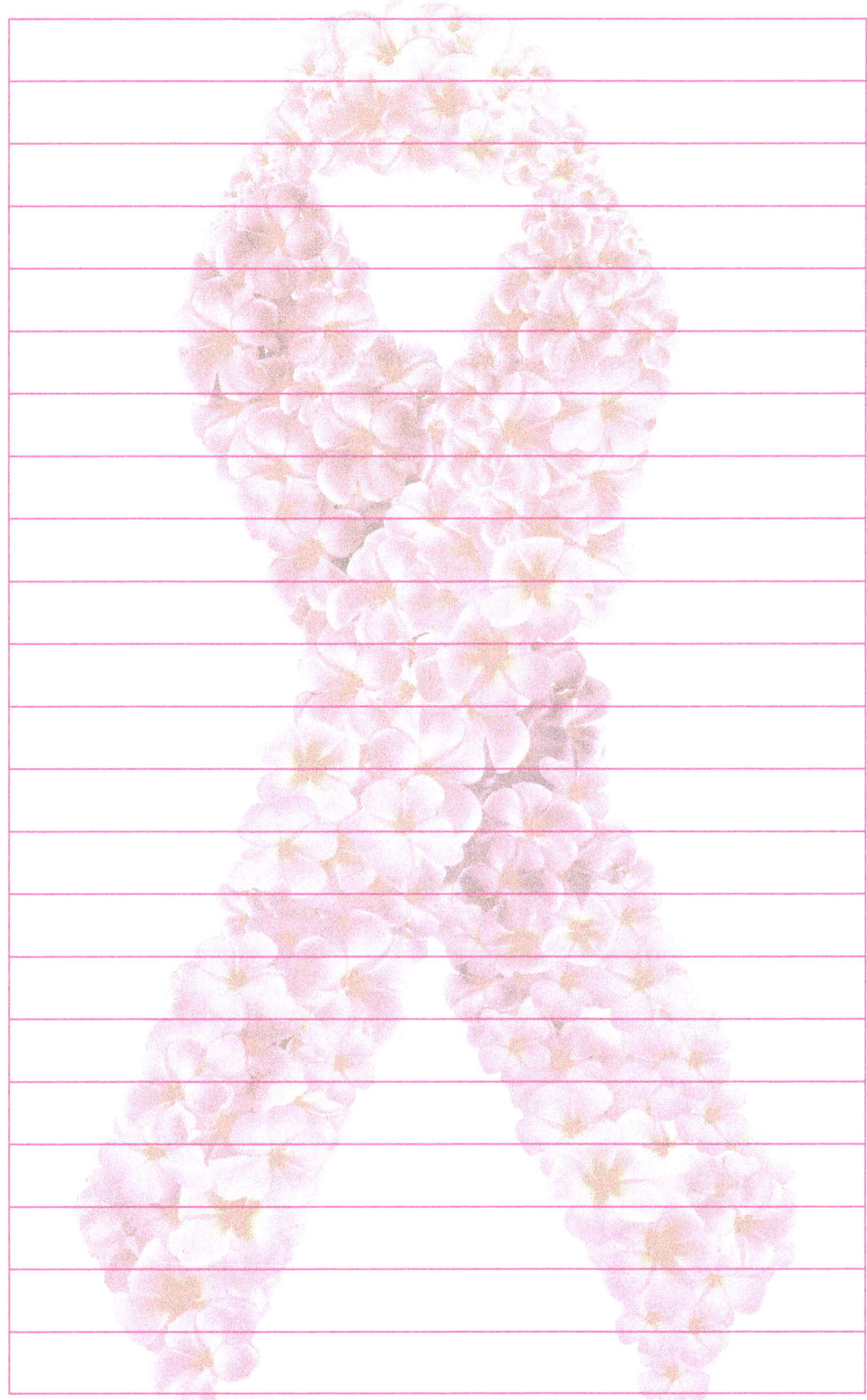

Date: _____ 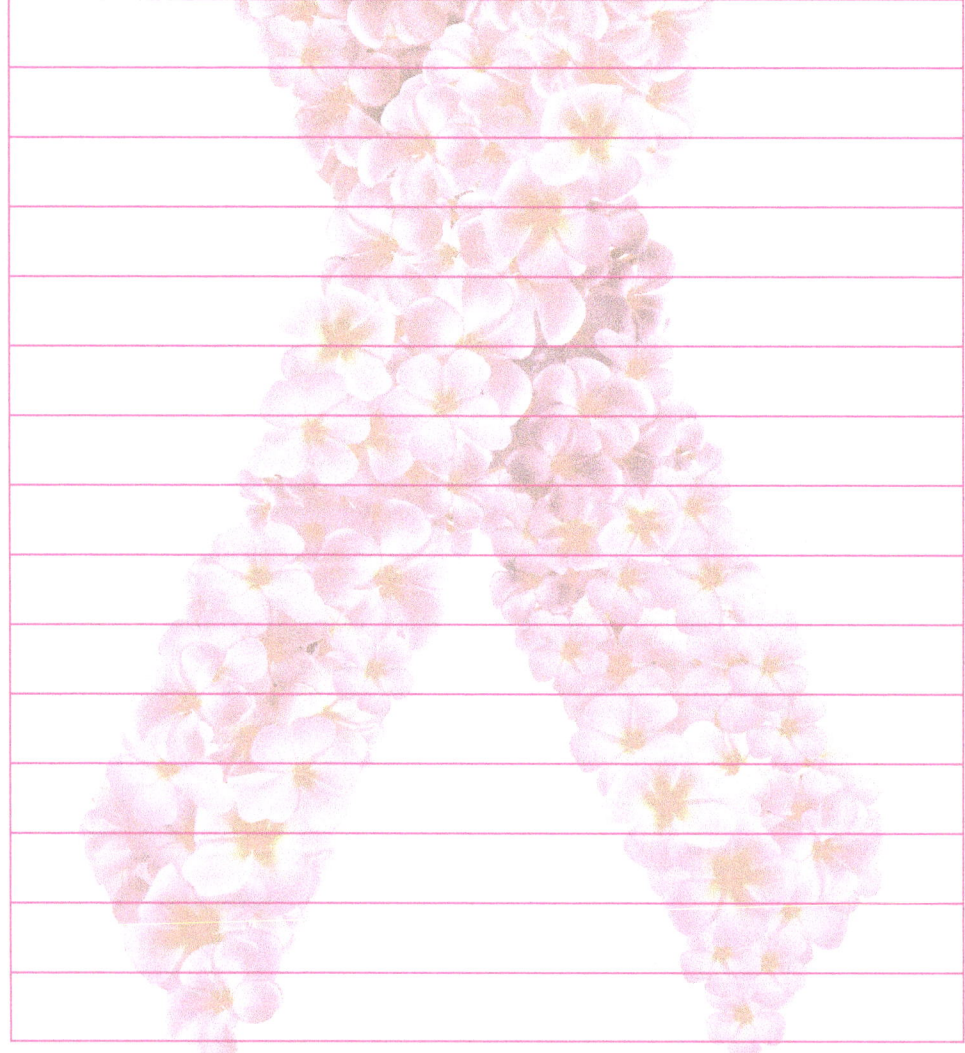 **Day 25**

Casting all your care upon him;
for he careth for you.
-1 Peter 5:7 KJV

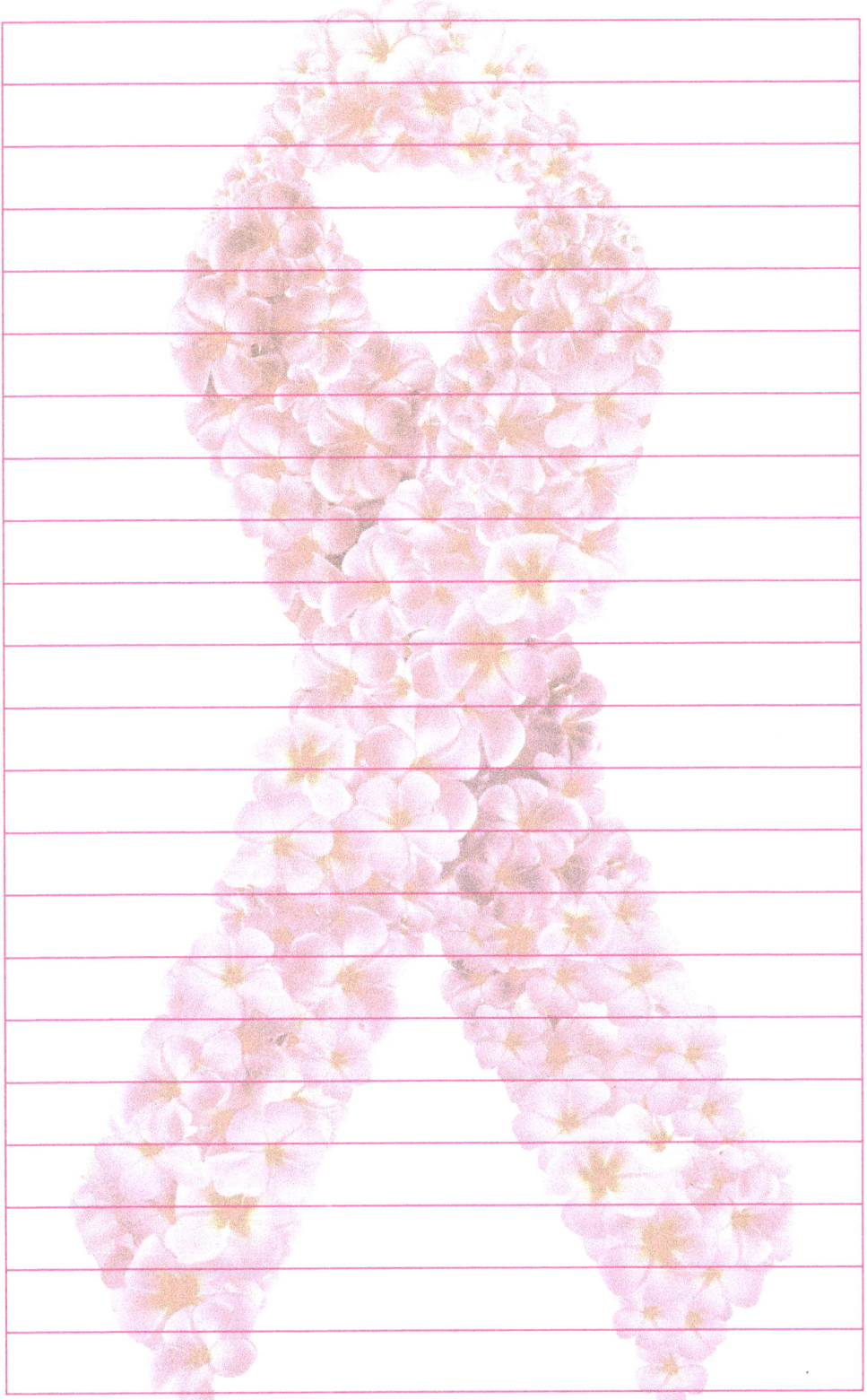

Date: _____ **Day 26**

And he who searches our hearts knows
the mind of the Spirit, because the Spirit
intercedes for God's people in
accordance with the will of God.
-Romans 8:27 NIV

Date: _____ **Day 27**

The Lord sustains them on their
sickbed and restores them
from their bed of illness.
-Psalm 41:3 NIV

77

Date: _____ **Day 28**

Trust in the Lord with all your heart,
And lean not on your own
understanding; in all your
ways acknowledge Him,
And He shall direct your paths.
-Proverbs 3:5-6

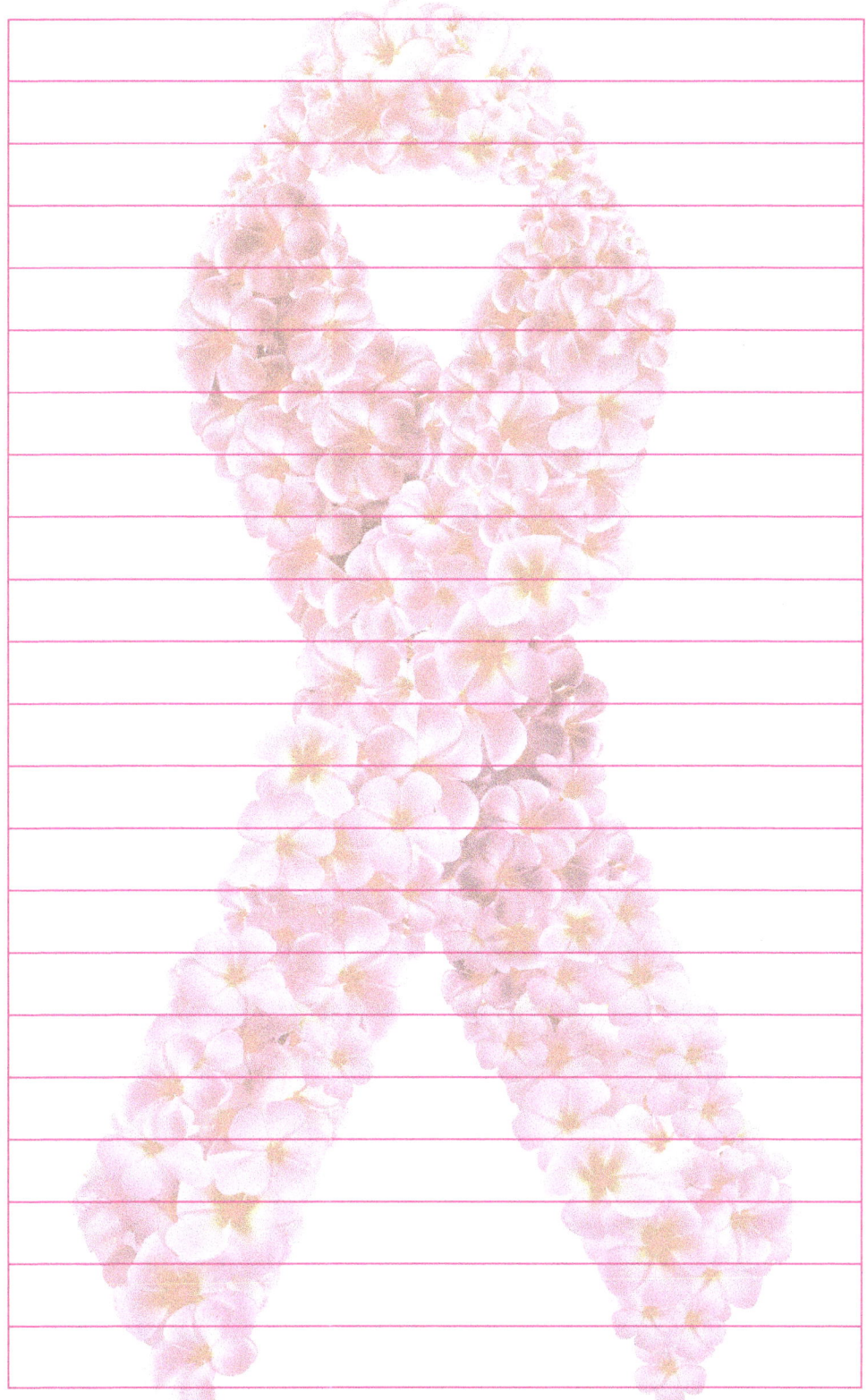

Date: _____ ## Day 29

But he said to me, "My grace is sufficient
for you, for my power is made perfect in
weakness." Therefore I will boast all the
more gladly about my weaknesses,
so that Christ's power may rest on me.
-2 Corinthians 12:9 NIV

Date: _____ **Day 30**

Finally, brethren, whatsoever things
are true, whatsoever things are honest,
whatsoever things are just, whatsoever
things are pure, whatsoever things are
lovely, whatsoever things are of good
report; if there be any virtue, and if there
be any praise, think on these things.
-Philippians 4:8 KJV

Date: _____ **Day 31**

[We pray that you may be]
strengthened and invigorated
with all power, according to His
glorious might, to attain every kind
of endurance and patience with joy,
-Colossians 1:11 AMP

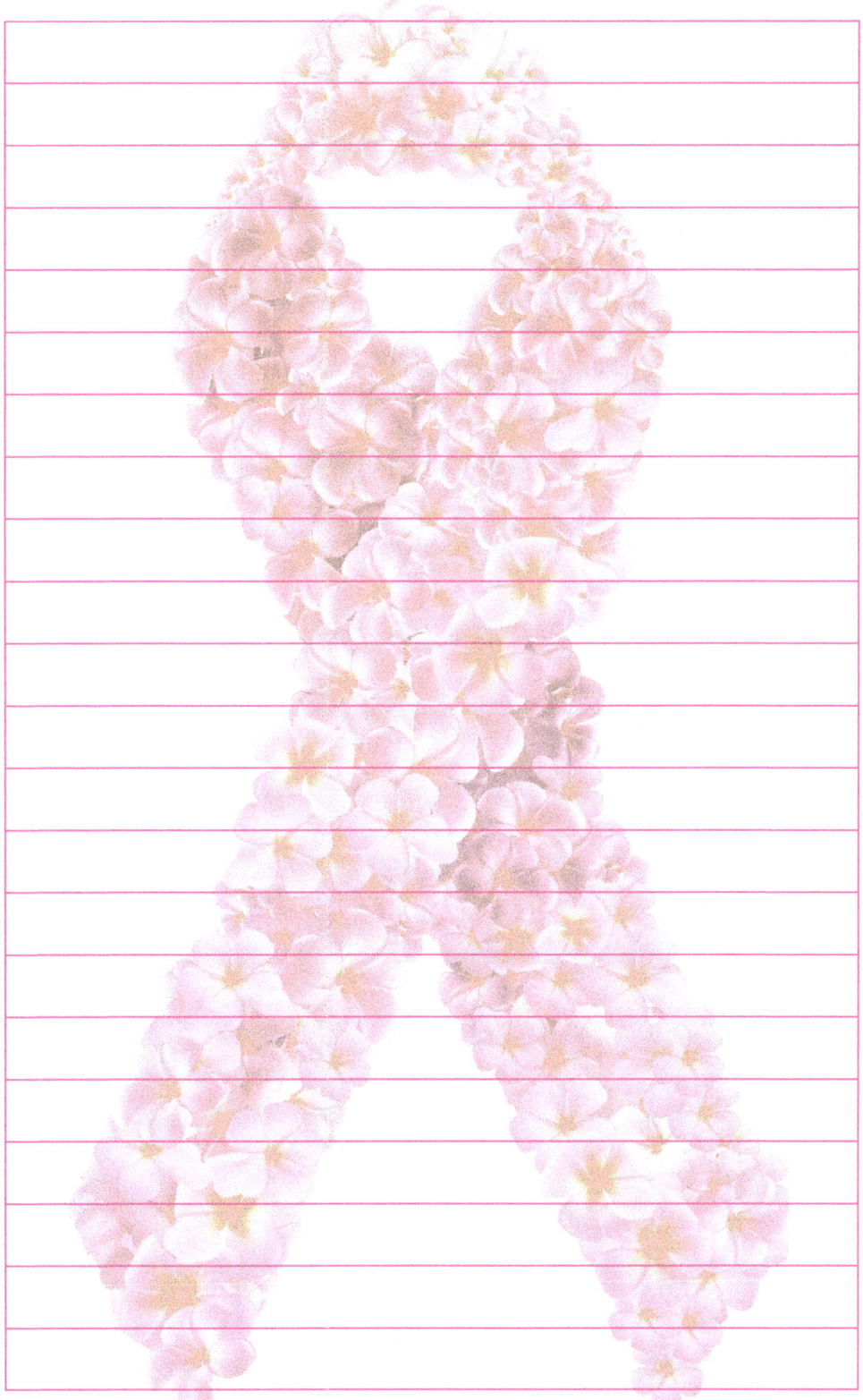

Date: _____ **Day 32**

He giveth power to the faint;
and to them that have no might
he increaseth strength.
-Isaiah 40:29 KJV

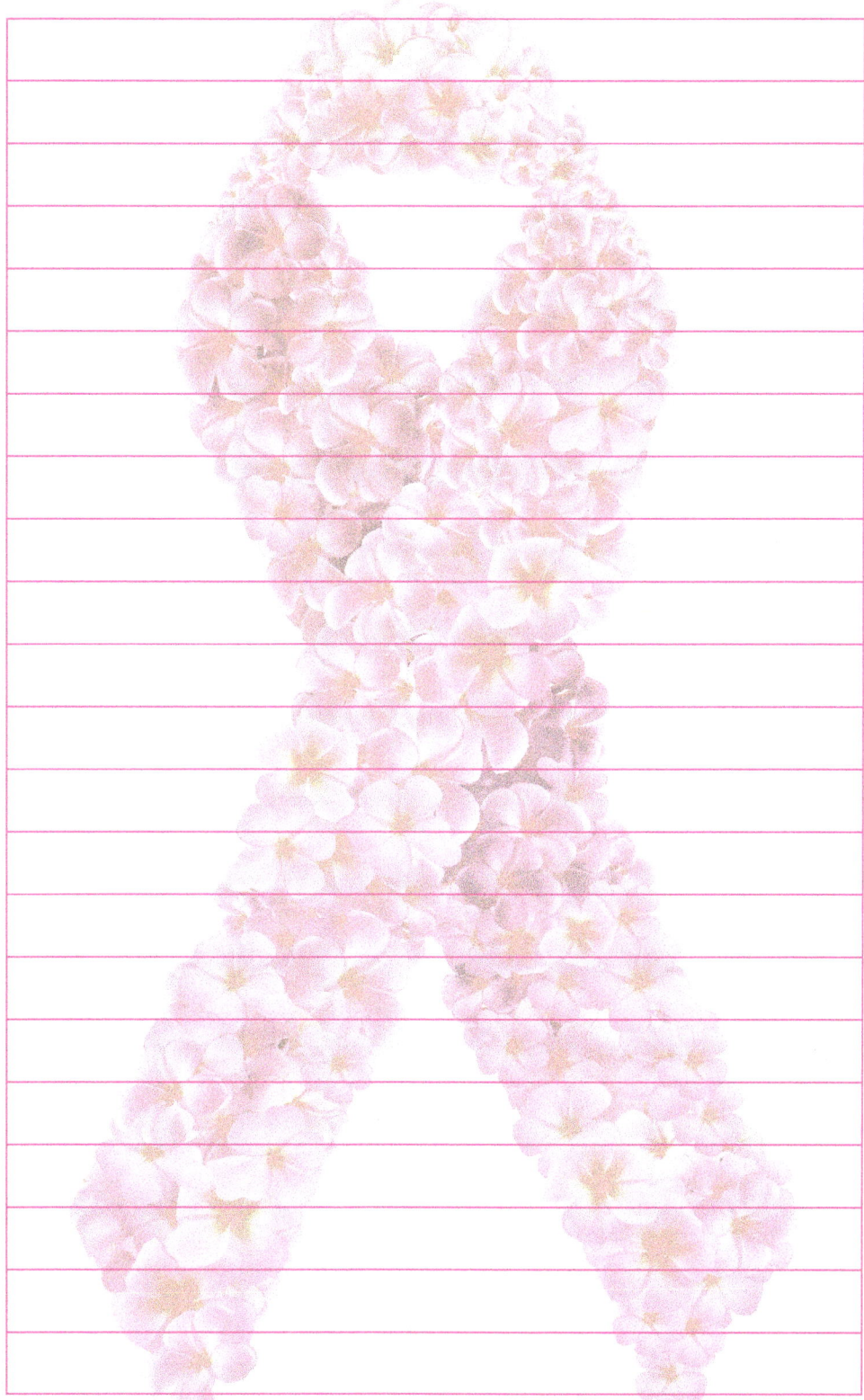

Date: _____ ## Day 33

Therefore we do not lose heart.
Though outwardly we are wasting away,
yet inwardly we are being renewed
day by day. For our light and momentary
troubles are achieving for us an eternal
glory that far outweighs them all.
-2 Corinthians 4:16-17 NIV

Date: _____ ## Day 34

[B]ut those who hope in the Lord
will renew their strength.
They will soar on wings like eagles;
they will run and not grow weary,
they will walk and not be faint.
-Isaiah 40:31 NIV

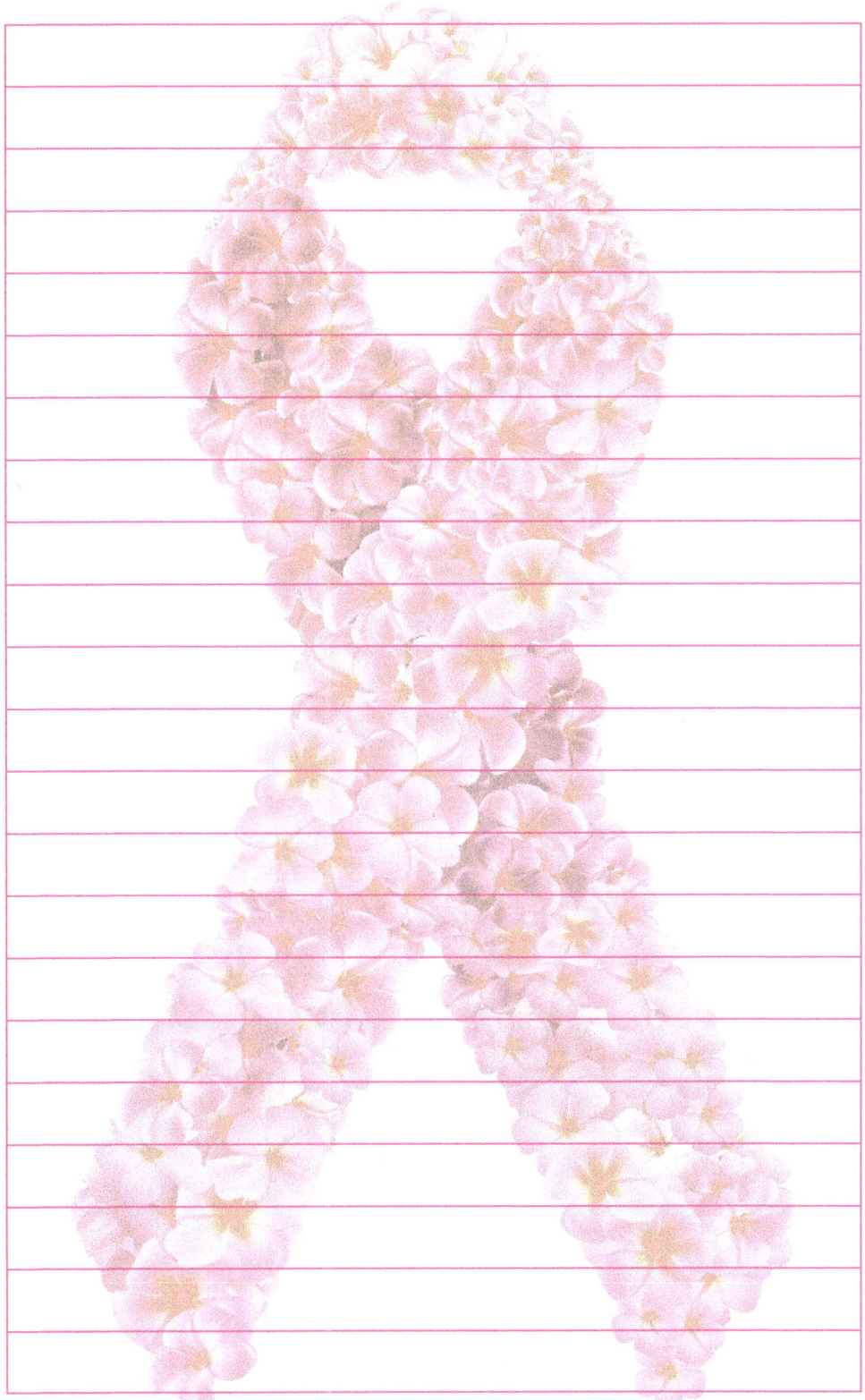

Date: _____ **Day 35**

In my distress I called to the Lord;
I cried to my God for help.
From his temple he heard my voice;
my cry came before him, into his ears.
-Psalm 18:6 NIV

Date: _____ **Day 36**

In my distress I cried unto the Lord,
and he heard me.
-Psalm 120:1 KJV

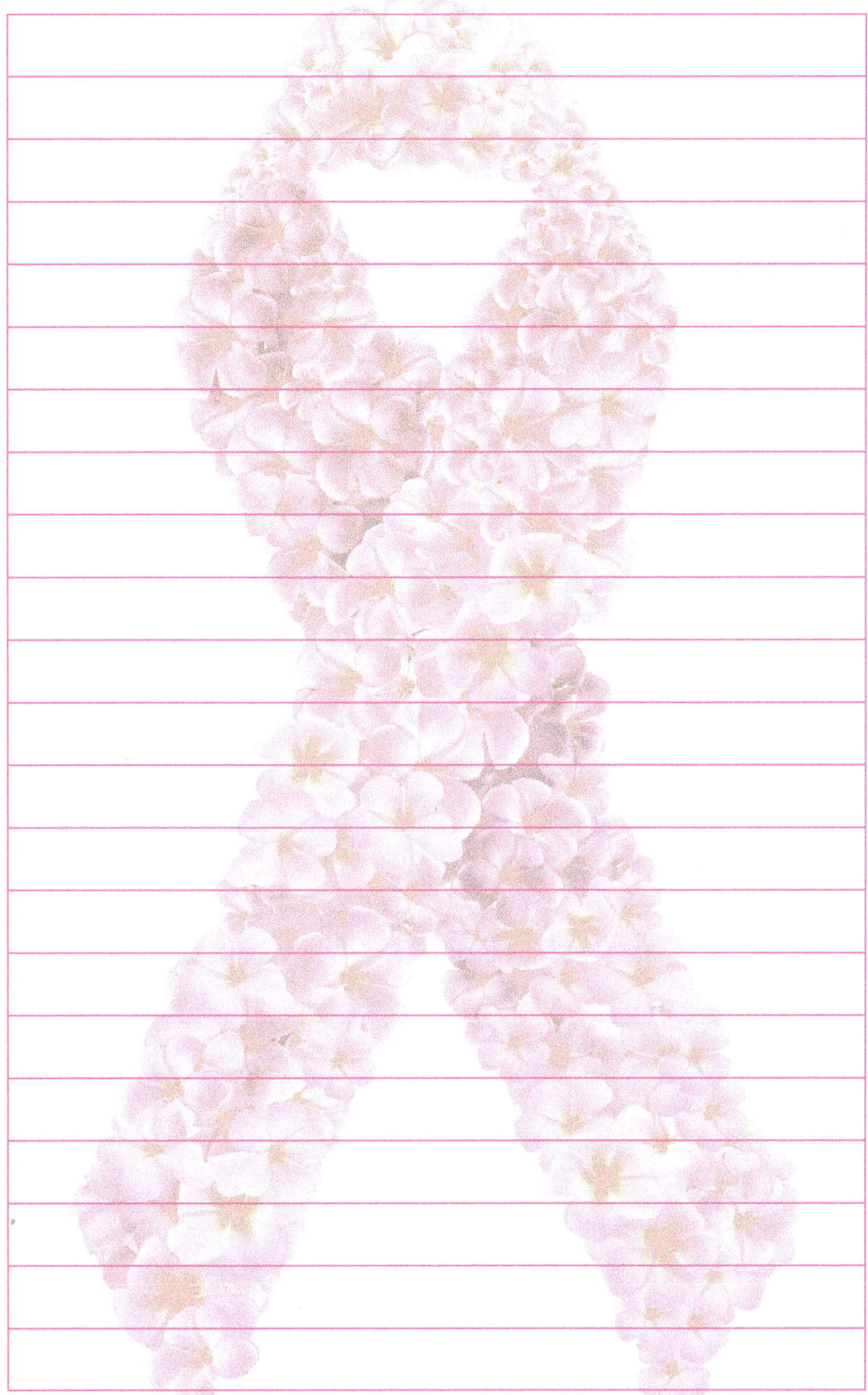

Date: _____ **Day 37**

Jesus looked at them and said,
"With man this is impossible,
but not with God;
all things are possible with God."
-Mark 10:27 NIV

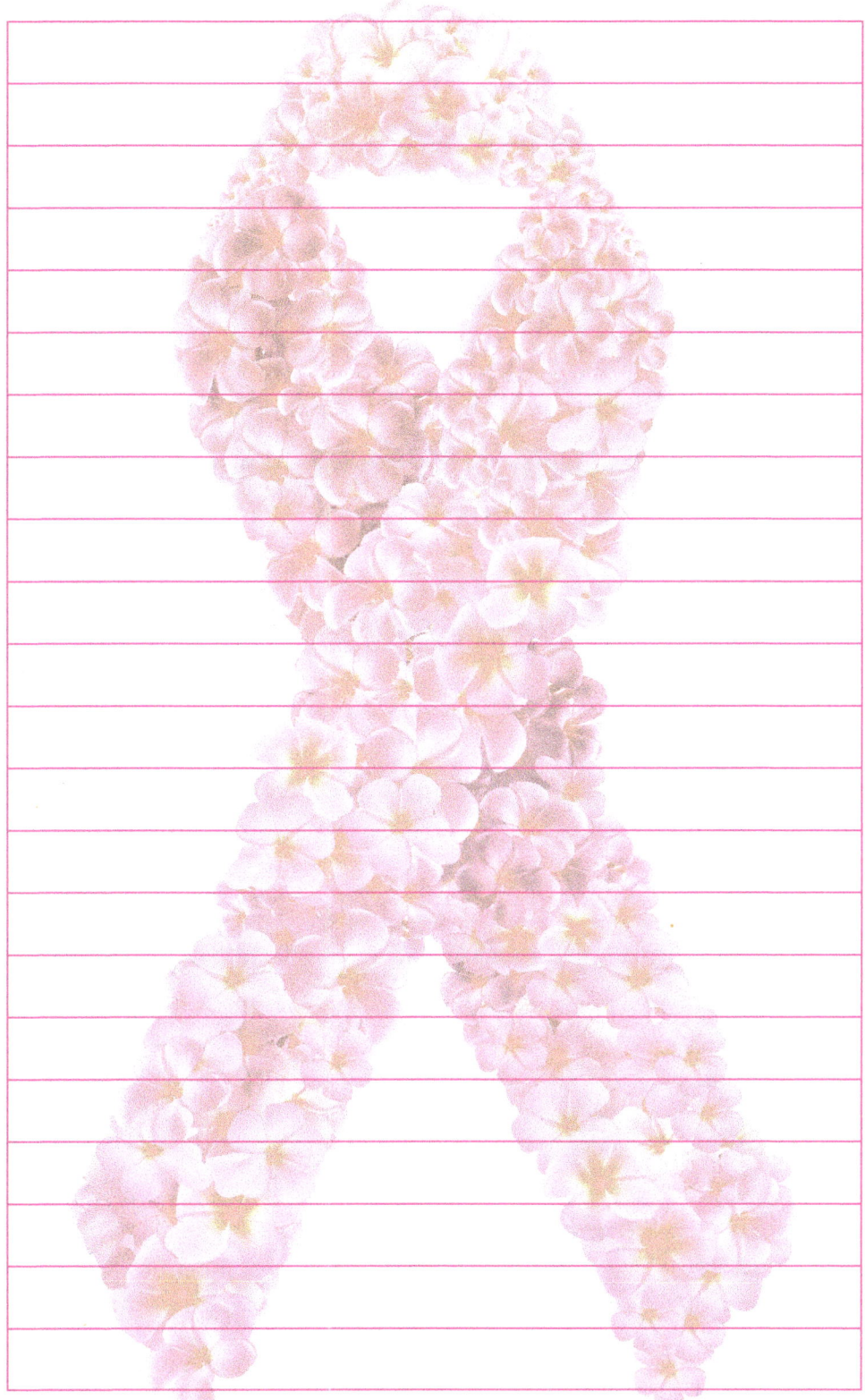

Date: _____ **Day 38**

["]Have I not commanded you?
Be strong and courageous.
Do not be afraid; do not be discouraged,
for the Lord your God will be
with you wherever you go."
-Joshua 1:9 NIV

Date: _____ **Day 39**

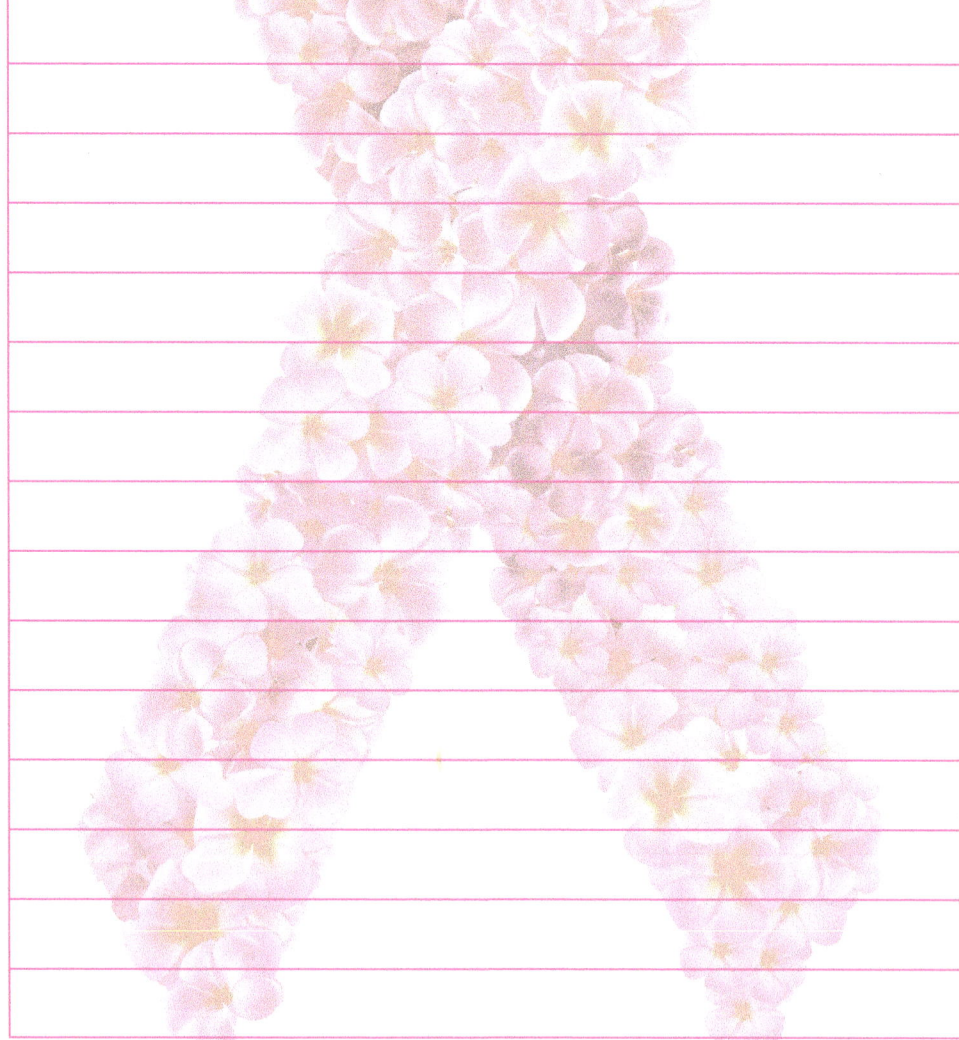

And ye shall seek me, and find me, when ye
shall search for me with all your heart.
-Jeremiah 29:13 KJV

Date: _____ **Day 40**

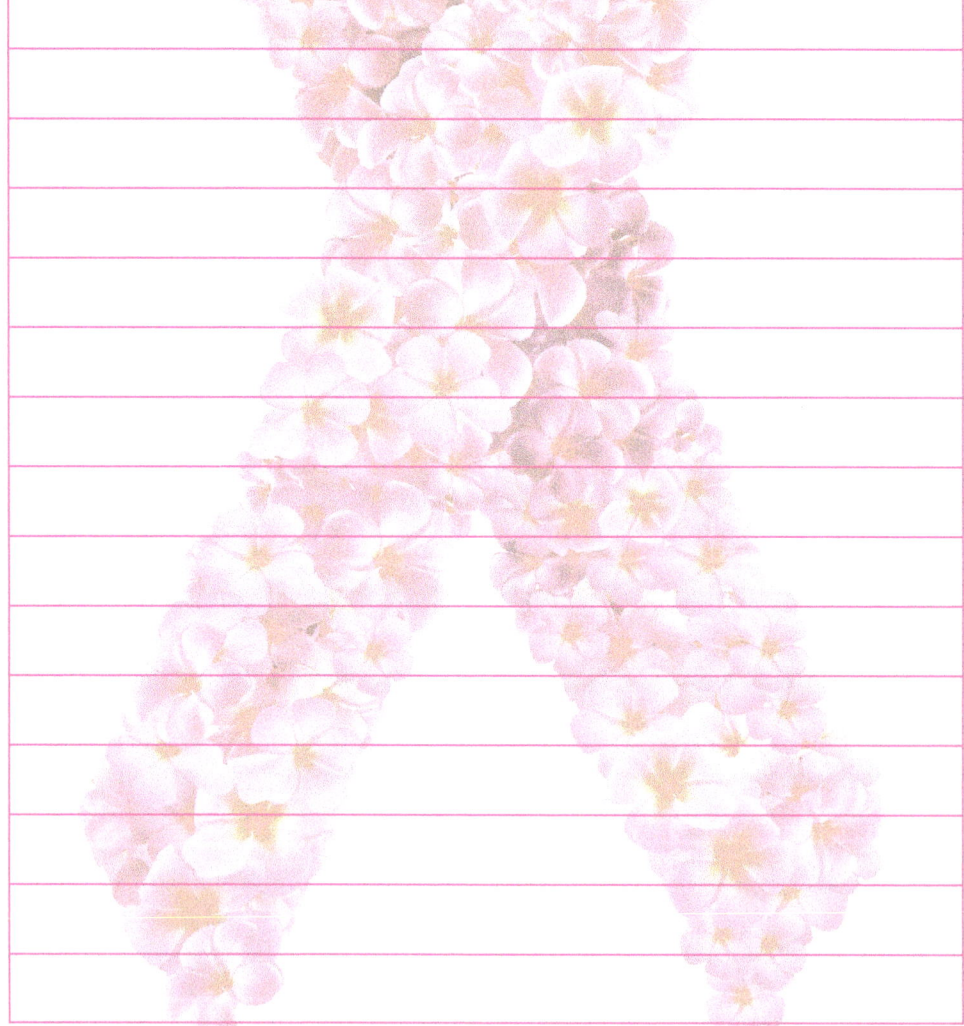

Rejoice in the Lord always:
and again I say, Rejoice.
-Philippians 4:4 KJV

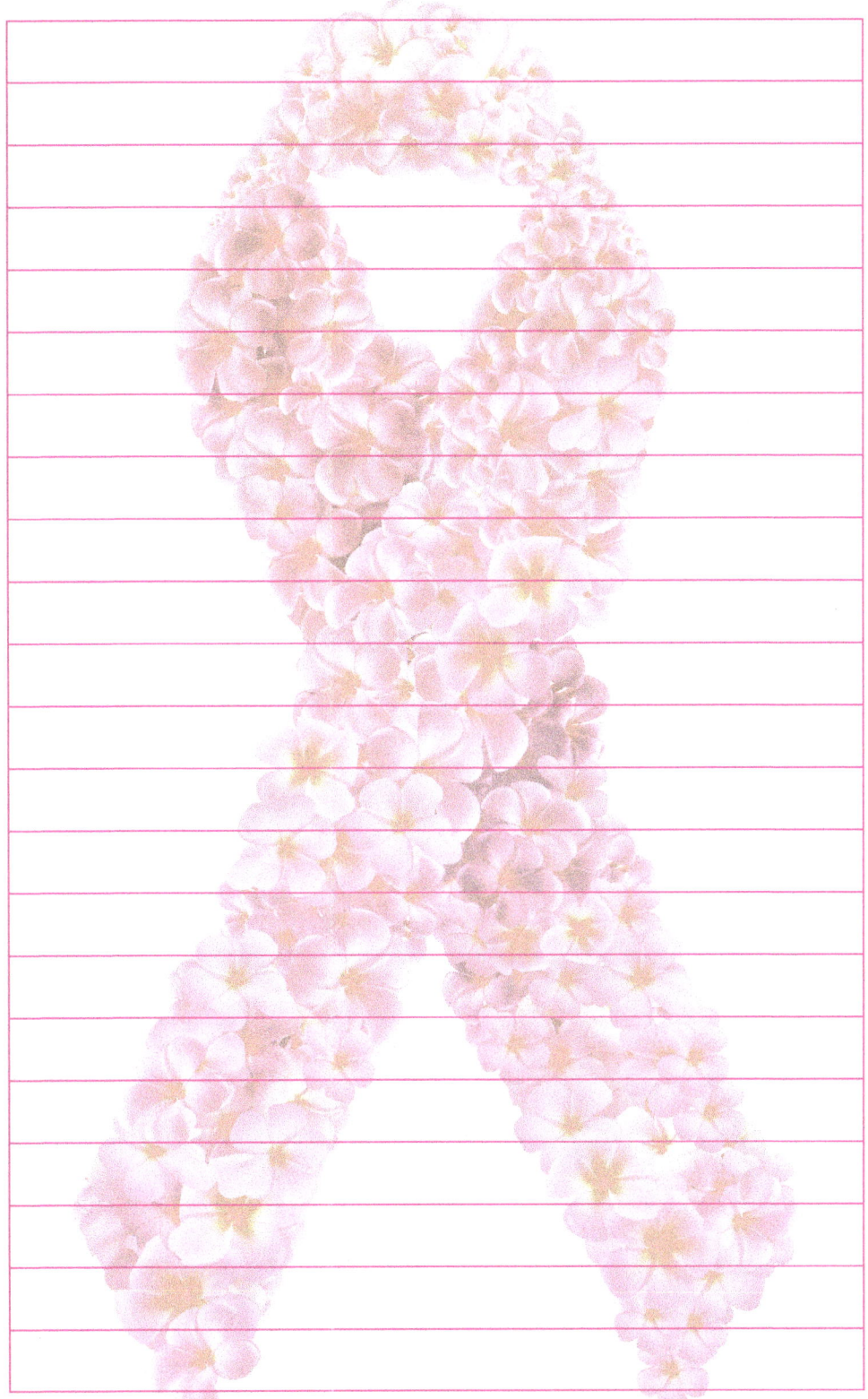

Testimonies
of Others

Earlene   107

Carissa   108

Earlene

Nothing could have prepared me for those chilling words: **"We see suspicious masses in three locations inside your left breast."** My emotions instantly swung from happy anticipation to absolute shock. *But I get a mammogram every year, and everything has always been fine,* I thought, struggling to comprehend the diagnosis. I was devastated.

I remember someone telling me that my journey wasn't just for me—it was meant to help someone else. At that moment, I desperately wished I could help others without having to face surgery, chemotherapy, radiation, and years of medication.

It was during the month of **October,** Breast Cancer Awareness Month, that I saw **sorors** in my chapter—all survivors—presented with gifts, celebrating the battles they had successfully fought. Initially, I was terrified to tell anyone, wanting to keep my diagnosis a secret. But the fear, combined with a powerful need for a confidante who understood my upcoming battle, weighed heavily on me. I found a trusted outlet in **Bonita Anderson**. The moment I told her about my breast cancer diagnosis, she offered a profound sense of peace. With a big, bright smile and a wonderfully calming voice, she simply said, **"It is okay, and you will be alright."** Hallelujah! In that instant, I knew I had a trusted ally who would walk with me through my journey.

Bonita's most important piece of advice—which I held onto throughout my treatment—was to **always be nice to the nurses and doctors**. I kept that in mind through two biopsies, a port insertion, two surgeries to remove the cancer, eight grueling rounds of chemotherapy, and thirty-three sessions of radiation.

Through it all, Bonita's smile and encouraging words were a vital source of inspiration and hope. I can never thank her enough for her guidance and support.

Carissa

Cancer? The National Cancer Institute (NCI) defines cancer as "a disease in which some of the body's cells grow uncontrollably and spread to other parts of the body".[1] According to World Health Organization (WHO) report in 2022, "there were approximately 20 million new cancer cases and nearly 9.7 million cancer deaths worldwide. WHO predicts that the number of cases will increase to 35 million by 2050, primarily due to population growth. Prevention efforts, such as avoiding tobacco use, eating a healthy diet, and maintaining a healthy weight, are crucial to reducing the future burden." [2]

[1]National Cancer Institute. "What Is Cancer?" *National Cancer Institute*, National Institutes of Health, 11 Oct. 2021, www.cancer.gov/about-cancer/understanding/what-is-cancer retrieved 10/14/25.

[2]World Health Organization. "World Health Organization." Who.int, World Health Organization, 2025, www.who.int/.

"We received your lab results.
It shows that you have cancer."

A medical professional telling you that you have cancer of any form is life-altering. It sure was for me. June 10, 2022 will forever be etched in my memory. Endometrial Cancer was the diagnosis. The antidote was the Biblical verse, "I shall not die, but live, and declare the works of the LORD" (Psalm 118:17), that I heard from the LORD on January 22, 2022 which resonated on D-day. So, I knew it was time to war for the prophecy and fulfillment of the word over my life.

Before I began my treatment, I contacted everyone I knew who had heard the dreadful words. But they had to be someone who I thought wouldn't tell everyone else. I wanted it to be kept a secret because I have found that when people hear "cancer" they automatically think of mortality. However, the LORD knew I would need my Childhood Friend and Sister to assist me to fight stronger together to be an overcomer.

Bonita Anderson – Woman of GOD, Wife, Mother, Grandmother, Daughter, Sister, Aunt, Friend, Community Activist, Nurse, Educator and Breast Cancer Warrior – has allowed her pain to become purpose. She is unashamed to let people know that she is a survivor. A person who is willing to share her truths about cancer. Bonita balances both her personal and professional knowledge of the disease to provide hope for others when rationality has momentarily ceased. She serves as a Pahokee (and Glades Area) pillar of strength demonstrating that there is still life to live even when you have been diagnosed with cancer. Even while going through treatment, she had perfect attendance at Lakeside Hospital. This display of resiliency allowed her to be awarded Nurse of the Year. Every seminar, training, event, or walk that Mrs. Anderson does is to provide awareness, promote screening as well as early detection, and informed decision-making regarding breast cancer.

My Sister, Bonita, was the notebook that I needed during a pivotal time to survive in the midst of a diagnosis. I'm excited about this journal that she has created! It is a part of her GOD-given ministry to help you, or someone you love, to navigate the discovery of cancer.

-Carissa, Cancer Free Since 2022

Your Personal Testimony

But may the God of all grace,
who called us to His eternal glory by
Christ Jesus, after you have suffered a while,
perfect, establish, strengthen, and settle you.
-1 Peter 5:10

Remember to write it down,
so you will always know your why!

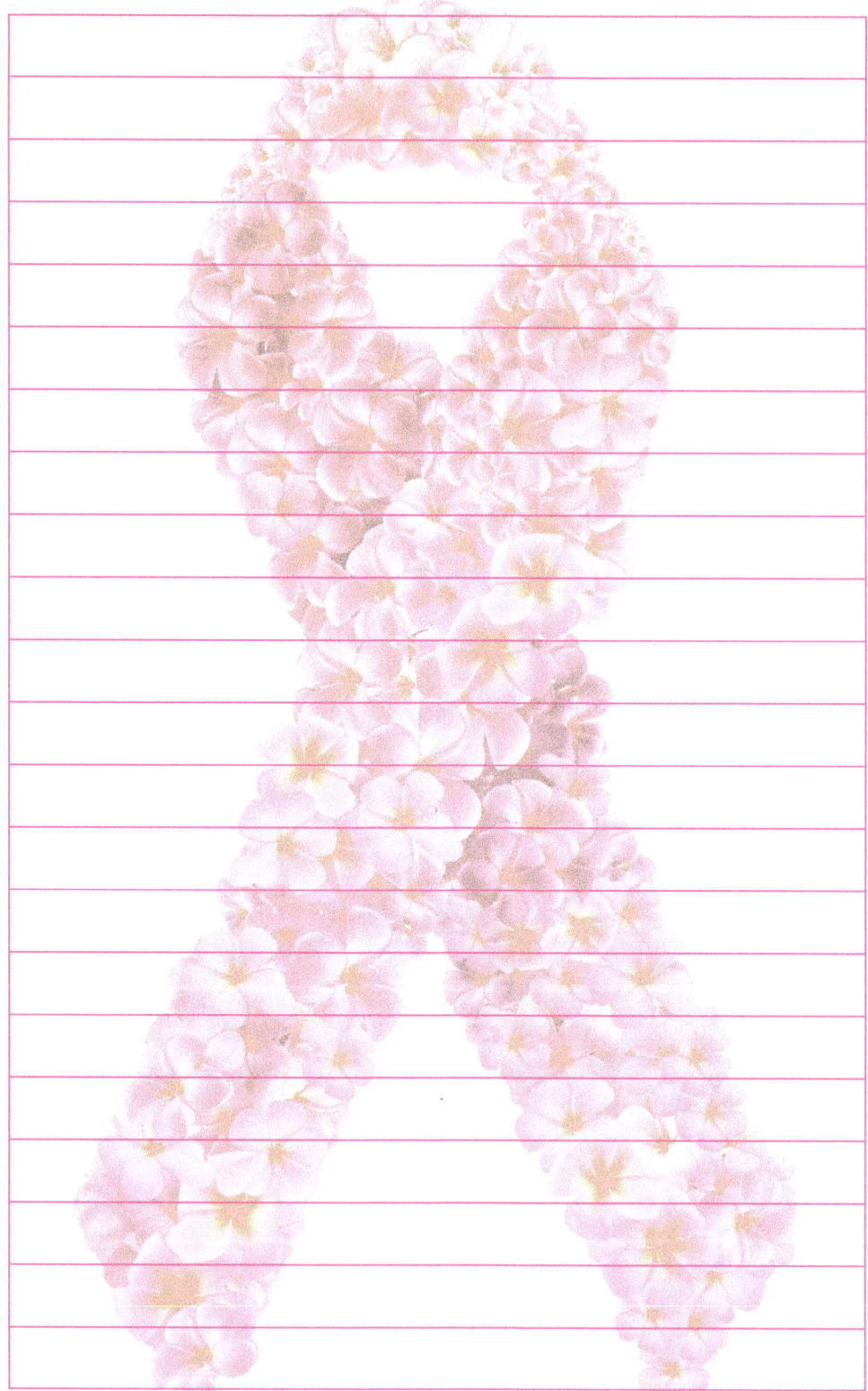

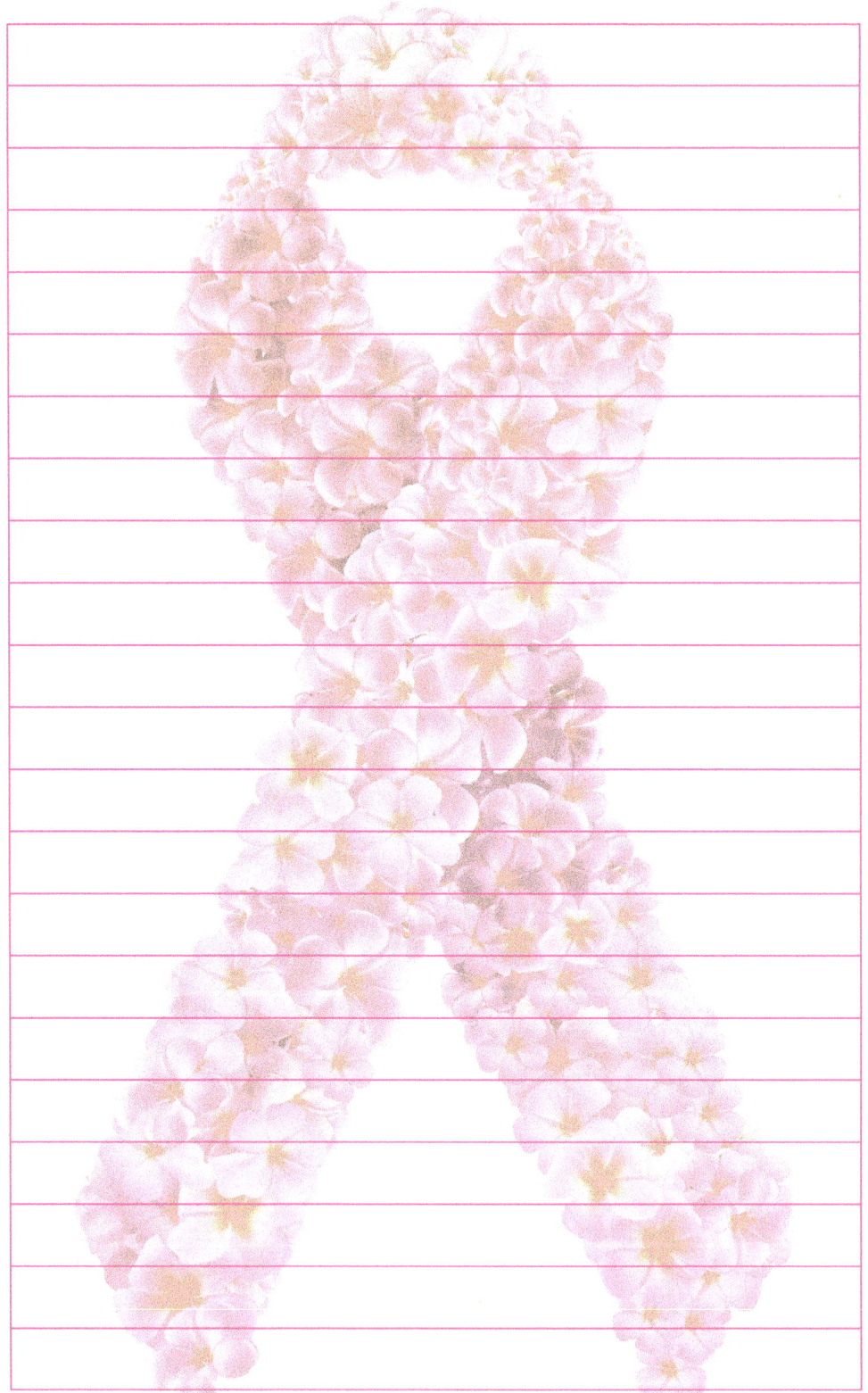

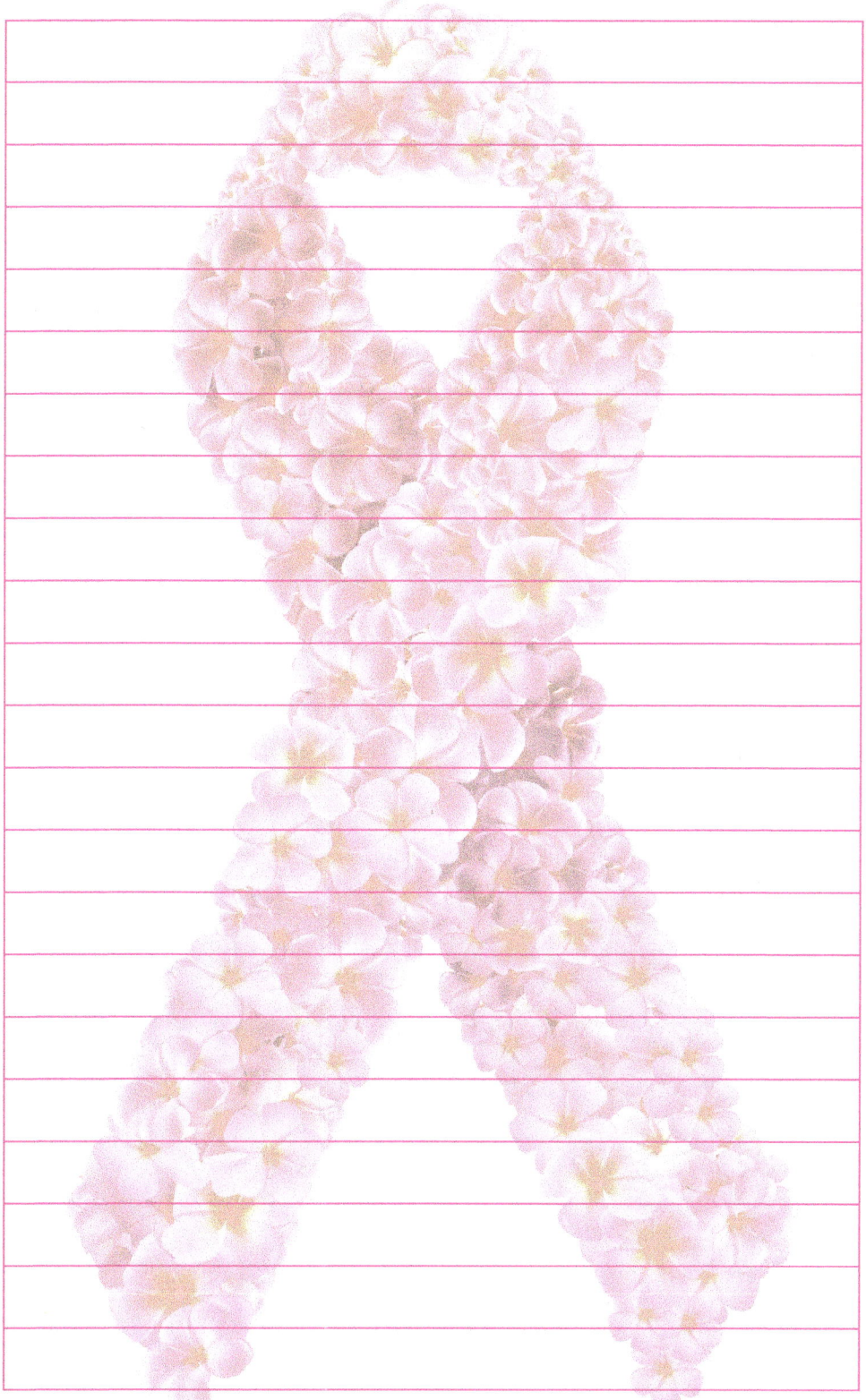

www.ingramcontent.com/pod-product-compliance
Lightning Source LLC
Chambersburg PA
CBHW051215120626
46547CB00013B/1357